PASS YOUR OB/GYN BOARD EXAM!

Fifth Edition

• How to Prepare for it • How to Take it • How to Pass It!

Anita Krishna Das, MD FACOG

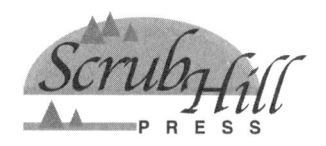

Scrub Hill PRESS

Copyright © 2016 by Anita Krishna Das, MD.
All rights reserved.

Publisher's Cataloging-in-Publication Data
Das, Anita Krishna.
Pass your Oral Ob/Gyn Board Exam! / Anita Krishna Das, MD, FACOG.

p. cm.
ISBN: 978-0-9822921-9-8

1. Obstetrics—Examinations, questions, etc. 2. Gynecology—Examinations, questions, etc.
R834.5 .D37 2009
618—dc22

Reproduction and translation of any part of this work beyond that permitted by Sections 107 and 108 of the United States Copyright Act without the permission of the copyright owners is unlawful.

The author and publisher have made every effort in the preparation of this book to ensure the accuracy of the information. However, the information in this book is sold without warranty, either express or implied. Neither the author nor Scrub Hill Press will be liable for any damages caused or alleged to be caused directly, indirectly, incidentally, or consequentially by the information in this book.

The opinions expressed in this book are solely those of the author and are not necessarily those of Scrub Hill Press.

Trademarks: Names of products mentioned in this book known to be a, or suspected of being trademarks or service marks are capitalized. The usage of a trademark or service mark in this book should not be regarded as affecting the validity of any trademark or service mark.

Publisher: Scrub Hill Press, Inc.
Interior Design: Shawn Morningstar
Editorial Assistance: Gloria Filebark

10 9 8 7 6 5 4 3 2

Scrub Hill PRESS

Arlington, VA 22204
800-516-1088
www.scrubhill.com

*This book is dedicated to
the thousands of oral exam
candidates that I have had the
joy, privilege and honor of mentoring.*

Table of Contents

Chapter 1
The Oral Versus the Written Exam: How They Differ 1

Chapter 2
The Application Process 5
    Applying for the Exam: Fast Track vs. Traditional 5
    Requirements 7
    Notification of Acceptance 7
    Limitations 8
    Qualifications 8

Chapter 3
Scope of the Exam 9

Chapter 4
Getting Started 11
    Priority of Study Topics 11
    References 12
    Review Courses 14
    Tutorial Courses 18
    Milestones 20

Chapter 5
The Case List   29

    Significance of the Exam   29
    Criteria for Admission to the Exam   30
    Collection of the Case List   31
    Initial Draft: Case-by-Case Entry   33
    List of Obstetric Patients   33
    Clinical Summary   41
    Initial ABOG Form Entry   41
    Clinical Summary   46
    Initial ABOG Form Entry   47
    List of Office Patients   47
    Clinical Summary—Conservative   53
    Clinical Summary—Speculative   53
    Peer Review   54
    Case List Logistics   55
    Strategic Organization of the Case List   57
    Editing   63
    Using the Case List as a Study Tool   66
    Defending Your Case List   67

Chapter 6
Kodachromes   101

Chapter 7
Case of the Day   105

Chapter 8
Studying for the Exam   117

    Mock Oral Exams   133

Chapter 9
Image Enhancement   **137**

Chapter 10
The Oral Exam   **141**

   The Day Before   142
   The Morning of the Exam   143
   Exam Content   144
   Exam Format   145
   Evaluation Criteria   146
   Examiner Alerts   146
   Exam Conduct   147
   Points for Style   151
   The End   153

Chapter 11
Test Results   **155**

   If You Fail…   157

Chapter 12
A Candidate's Journey   **161**

Chapter 13
Lessons Learned   **175**

Appendix A
ABOG Acceptable Case List Abbreviations   **183**

Appendix B
Acronyms and Abbreviations   **185**

Appendix C
Addresses   **187**

Appendix D
Custom Case List   189

ABOG Software   189
Commercial Software   190
Customized Case List   191
Paradigm Shift   191
Software   192
Setting Up Your Own Database   196
Setting Up Your Obstetric Database   203
Setting Up Your Gynecologic Database   205
Setting Up Your Office Practice Database   205

Appendix E
Recommendations for Subspecialty Fellows   211

Appendix F
Recommendations for Military Personnel   215

Appendix G
Case List Review   217

Index   219

Preface

The failure of one of our glowing junior faculty members to pass his oral OB/GYN board exam scared me into thinking about the exam the last year of my residency. I knew I was going to practice in a town remote from an academic center, so I figured I had better get all the help I could while still under the protective cloak of a knowledgeable faculty.

My bubble was burst. I asked everyone, and they hardly knew anything about the exam. I couldn't find much on the subject matter (other than "Know everything"), the process ("I've repressed all of that"), or the conduct of the exam ("They grill you under the hot white lights"). Logically, I turned to graduates who had recently taken the exam. The little bit of information I unearthed was inconsistent.

I was worried, but life got busy with finishing residency, moving and joining a practice. I was hopeful that my uneasiness would wane after I began the process and my worries would be for naught. I was wrong. The ABOG guidelines were vague and generic. I was lost and overwhelmed about how or where to begin.

I dedicated a year and a half to preparing for the exam. Life got put on hold. I have never prepared so hard for a test. But I was ready.

During the exam, I knew my stuff. Yet the examiners were skilled at leaving a fragment of doubt with most questions. By the end of the exam, I didn't know if I had passed. I was outraged. I knew I really knew my stuff, and no one deserved to pass more than me. Fortunately, I received my congratulatory letter in just three days, so I was not in agony for long. As I read the letter, I was flooded with relief, but then my anger began to swell. I threw down the letter and cried, "There has to be a better way."

I had learned so much about the process of preparing for and taking the exam that I felt compelled to share it. Fortuitously, the medical school in the state where I practiced did not have an OB/GYN residency, so I linked up with a national review course. As I shared my experiences throughout the country, two things happened. The first was that I was able to tap into the target audience and accumulate a huge pool of feedback about exam experiences. Second, because there are so few resources on the topic, I was inundated with appreciation and encouraged to make this information more widely available.

This fifth edition updates recent numerous changes in exam topics and format. There is a continued trend toward standardizing the test. Currently, the exam consists of only the case list and the structured cases. Standardization in general has made a debut with ACOG practice check lists. Simulation labs enable us to practice what we preach and I predict may someday be incorporated as a means of certification and credentialing, also. The Maintenance of Certification (MOC) process also puts us all on the same sheet of music. Although you do not start this process until after you pass your oral boards, the fact that ABOG chooses the articles is free insight as to what topics they consider important.

Interesting that this fifth edition already reflects the pendulum swinging back toward the philosophy in the first edition, in that finally we're back to being specialists rather than primary care doctors. However, that pendulum has over swung, as we've become even more sub-specialized with laborists, intensivists and hospitalists. Additionally, 2013 marked the official recognition of Female Pelvic Medicine and Reconstructive Surgery as the fourth boarded sub specialty, pushing many generalists out of Urogynecology.

The rapidly evolving climate in the business of medicine has impacted us as well. At least half of physicians are now employees rather than private practitioners. This impacts the depth and breadth of our practice, and extends into our exam preparation as well. Whereas in the past, board certification was a feather in your cap, now it's almost mandatory in order to practice. Most hospital privileges and insurance reimbursements are contingent upon being board certified.

In 2012, ABOG implemented their Test Integrity Policy (TIP). TIP restricts disclosing specific exam questions. This fifth edition reflects compliance with their request.

This fifth edition also marks twenty five years of my mentoring physicians seeking their board certification. I marvel that the approach recommended in the first edition has stood the test of time. Of course, I have fine-tuned it throughout the years, but this approach is really quite simple, and perhaps that's the reason for its success.

Preface

This book will help you to organize and prioritize your studies, but you will still have to roll up your sleeves and learn the stuff cold. Please consider most carefully my advice on how to construct your case list. A well-constructed case list makes all the difference in its defense. This book will also reduce your anxiety about taking the exam, but you still have to practice, practice, practice with mock orals to get proficient with the oral exam format.

I am readily available to assist you throughout the entire process. You may contact me at krisdas@americasboardreview.com or 1-877-ABC- OBGYN.

I hope this book is a compass for you. May it give you the shortest and easiest path to board certification. Good luck!

Krishna Das, MD, FACOG
February 2016

Chapter 1

The Oral Versus the Written Exam: How They Differ

The most common test format throughout medical school and residency is a written exam. Years of experience with the written format make taking your primary written exam straightforward and predictable. Preparing for and taking an oral exam, however, are quite different. Experimentation with the oral exam format should not be reserved for your first encounter with the oral boards.

The oral boards differ from the written boards in several ways. The first of which is timing. You cannot sit for the oral exam until you have successfully completed the written exam. Most graduates have transitioned into clinical practice, which is just enough time to fall out of the mandatory rigors of the academic environment of residency. No more morning report, morbidity and mortality conference, or grand rounds—just enough time to have succumbed to "the good life," just enough time to "get out of shape" for intense academic discipline. This academic apathy results in a rude awakening when you face the intensity of effort that will be required to prepare adequately for the oral exam.

Isolation from the medical center mecca not only predisposes to academic laxity, but also strips away the advantage of "misery loves company" that helps to motivate studying. Typically, residents prepare collectively for upcoming tests, such as CREOG (Council on Resident Education in Obstetrics and Gynecology) in-service exams and the written board exam.

Often there are even formal study groups; furthermore, staff mentors are eager to share knowledge gained from previous residents' experience. After all, the program's reputation is at stake. Poor performance on standardized tests is a reflection of the staff's mentoring. The group's efforts culminate in the written exam at the end of residency.

Upon graduation from residency and successful completion of the written boards, active candidates migrate to all corners of the country. Most join practices with senior partners who have already completed the oral exam process. Thus, the severing of academic ties strips away the familiar comfort of camaraderie as you tackle the oral exam.

For the first time, and unfortunately for the biggest test of our career, most of us have no idea of the format, let alone the test topics. The familiarity of a written exam is gone, and you are all alone. Most commonly, the residency programs do nothing to prepare you for what's to come. Thus, most of us lacked the foresight and insight during residency to tap into the faculty's knowledge about the oral exam. Most residents cannot, or refuse to, see past the written exam. After all, you can't even sit for the orals until you pass the written board exam.

So now you're isolated. Your partners and local colleagues can't remember (or have purposely repressed) the details you need. Your out-of-town resident colleagues don't know any more than you. The feeling of impending doom and panic sets in.

Yet the biggest obstacle of all is time. Everybody competes for your time. Residency is no longer an acceptable excuse. Family, social, civic, and church demands—let alone your practice—make finding time to prepare for the exam almost humanly impossible.

In addition to timing, another major difference between the oral and the written boards is format. The purpose of the written exam is to confirm a foundation of knowledge in the basic sciences. On the other hand, the oral exam confirms the ability to apply that basic knowledge to patient care.

Successful performance on the written exam is no guarantee for similar success with the oral exam. Unlike a written exam, regurgitation of isolated facts is not good enough. Furthermore, selection of the "right" answer is merely the beginning, not the end, in the oral exam. You must be able to substantiate your answers unhesitatingly.

Finally, the significance of "needing" to pass the oral exam has changed. Customarily, everyone has to take, but not pass, the written boards to graduate from residency. Thankfully, however, you don't have to be board-certified to practice medicine. Historically, board certification is a feather in your cap—a mark of prestigious academic excellence.

Thanks to managed care, hospital-owned practices, Joint Commission, and CMS, all of that has changed. Board certification is now required for participation in many insurance plans, hospital staff privileges, and practice employment. You can still practice medicine without board certification, but not necessarily how or where you want to practice. Thus, more is at stake with the oral exam—in fact, maybe everything.

In conclusion, the oral exam differs from the written exam in its timing, format and impact on your ability to practice medicine. The task of preparing for the oral board exam is enormous. There are no short cuts. As an anonymous philosopher observed, "The only place where success comes before work is in the dictionary." In contrast to the written exam, a photographic memory affords little advantage. Finally, hard work is rewarded. With the oral exam, you truly get out of it what you put into it. Testimonials from those who have failed repeatedly confirm this observation.

The task is surmountable. The entire elephant can be eaten, but only one bite at a time. The following chapters will tell you how to successfully eat that elephant. Get out your fork and knife, and come with a ravenous appetite. Bon appétit!

Chapter 2

The Application Process

Applying for the Exam: Fast Track vs. Traditional

The *Bulletin* published by the American Board of Obstetrics and Gynecology, Inc. is a guideline for the application process. This resource is invaluable and you will refer to it repeatedly throughout the entire process. You may download a copy from their website at **www.abog.org**.

Since 2002, candidates can apply for the accelerated oral exam process. Historically, you had to wait two years between successful completion of the written exam and the oral exam. In 2002, however, this was shortened to a one year wait between the two tests.

There are pros and cons for each track. The advantage of the fast track is you get it over with sooner. Why put off until tomorrow what you can do today? You also can ride on the academic momentum of your written exam preparation, rather than letting it slide away for another year.

The advantage of the traditional track is that it's logistically easier. You get a whole year to get settled into your new practice, community, lifestyle, etc. In the fast track, you have to begin collecting cases within a week after completing the written exam. Furthermore, the exponential growth in your clinical skills the first couple of years in practice will really help you on the exam. For these reasons, I recommend the traditional track.

I recommend the fast track only if you are immediately starting into a practice limited to just obstetrics or gynecology or you are planning to pursue subspecialty fellowship training. Since you are examined in both topics, you won't forget as much in one year. However, you will need to use cases from your chief year in the off subject. In other words, if you are planning a GYN-only practice, you will need to use obstetrical patients from your chief residency year for your obstetrics case list. Obviously, this will be a piece of cake if you are reading this in your residency and you now know to SAVE THAT CASE LOG! If you are having an "oops" moment and realize you gleefully pitched it when you were cleaning out the chief resident's desk, now is the time to make arrangements to recapture that data.

If you choose the "fast track," you must return your oral exam application sent with your written exam results (or go on-line to www.abog.org), along with your application fee by September 15th of the year preceding the oral exam. You will be notified by October 1st if you have been accepted into the accelerated process. Thereafter, you must meet the same requirements as the other candidates.

If you do not elect the fast track, the application form for the oral exam may be requested on-line at **www.abog.org**. Currently, the application is not available until February 1st. However, you will be defending cases from July 1st to June 30th. Do not delay those seven months until you apply, to begin collecting your cases, as you will be overwhelmingly behind. Thus, I recommend that you order your case list software in July or August, but certainly no later than September.

The completed application form, the application fee, a copy of each current medical license and the completed Hospital Privileges Verification form must be received on or before March 15th of the year of the exam. A late fee is charged for applications received between March 16th and April 15th—and an even steeper fee for applications received between April 16th and April 30th. No applications are accepted after April 30th. If your application (not necessarily your case list) is accepted, you will be notified in July. Once you are notified in July of your admissibility to the oral exam, you must send the examination fee and your case list and upload your digital identification photograph by August 1st. You can submit your case list as late as August 14th, but you will, of course, be assessed a late fee. No case lists or examination fees are accepted after August 15th.

Requirements

The ABOG *Bulletin* lists the requirements to sit for the exam. In addition you are accountable for the ABOG policies outlined online. Only the highlights are listed below:

1. You must have achieved a passing grade on the written exam taken no longer than five years before the oral exam.

2. You must report any and all negative actions taken against your license at any time, even if the action has been cleared or ended.

3. You must have an unrestricted license to practice medicine in the United States or its territories or a province of Canada since at least June 1st of the year preceding the exam. Candidates practicing in any other country must submit a letter from a senior officer of their hospital(s) verifying their credentials.

4. You must be actively engaged in an unsupervised practice, which is defined as: independent, continuous, unsupervised patient care *limited* to obstetrics and gynecology, from July 1st of the year preceding the exam through June 30th of the year of the exam. A maximum of 8 weeks of absence from practice for all reasons is allowed.

5. A practice that consists exclusively of ambulatory care is not considered adequate.

6. You must submit a case list.

Notification of Acceptance

You will be notified in July or October of the year of your exam if your application is accepted, as well as the month of your exam, for the traditional or fast track, respectively. You will also receive you case list ID # with this notification letter. You must then log in to your ABOG personal home page, pay the examination fee, and upload a current digital photograph. You must then submit your case list by August 1st, and if it is approved by the Board, you will receive an "Authorization for Admission" notifying you of the date and time of your exam approximately one month prior to your assigned examination week.

Limitations

You must pass the oral exam within six years of passing the written exam, unless serving in a board-approved fellowship. You may take the oral exam only three times. If you fail the oral exam three times or do not pass the oral exam within six years, you must repeat and pass the written exam before you can take the oral exam again. Effective in 2018, you must achieve board certification within 8 years of the completion of training.

Qualifications

The candidate must be of good moral and ethical character. Your character may be verified by inquiry to administrative officers of organizations and institutions to whom your mode of practice is known. Furthermore, time spent in a teaching or research position that does not provide sufficient evidence of independent, continuous and unsupervised responsibility for patient care is not permissible. Falsification of data (including case lists) or evidence of other "professional misbehavior" may result in deferral of a candidate's application for at least three years.

Chapter 3

Scope of the Exam

The purpose of the exam is to evaluate your knowledge and skills in solving clinical problems in obstetrics, gynecology and women's health. Most importantly, you are expected to demonstrate a level of competence that allows you to serve as a consultant to non-obstetrician-gynecologists in your community.

There is no better DNA of a practitioner's mode of practice than his case list. This is the one component of the exam that has remained constant for many years. Thus, half of your test is devoted to defending your case list. You must demonstrate the following abilities when questioned from your case list:

1. to develop a diagnosis, including the necessary clinical, laboratory and diagnostic procedures
2. to select and apply proper treatment under elective and emergency conditions
3. to prevent, recognize and manage complications
4. to plan and direct follow-up and continuing care

The *Bulletin* clearly states the case list is an essential component of the test. For years defending the case list has comprised half of your test. The other half has varied through the years. However, since 2007 the other half has been exclusively the structured cases.

This vague, yet all-encompassing subject matter makes studying rather challenging. In 2015, ABOG published a list of test topics in addition to the case list categories. Additionally, ABOG does not disclose their grading scale.

Their feedback to candidates who fail is characteristically noncommittal. The ABOG Diplomate states only that "the mode of practice continues to be the major reason for failure."

Don't despair, as your chances of passing the exam are excellent. ABOG reports that, since 1990, the pass rate for first time takers for all candidates, American or international graduates, is about 85%. These statistics, however, are skewed and falsely reassuring. Usually only the best-prepared candidates sit for the exam. Because most candidates have invested at least 16 months of preparation, they represent "survival of the fittest". Thus, only the best need apply—that is, until recently.

The advent of managed care and CMS' pay for performance will lead to a new set of statistics. Symbolically, board certification has been a prestigious badge of academic excellence. Such accolades, however, were not necessary to practice medicine—until now. Increasingly, only board-certified physicians are selected as providers for HMOs and similar insurance groups. Consequently, both hospitals and group practices are forced to require the same of their staff. Board certification has become mandatory to ensure financial livelihood.

As all comers begin to apply for the exam, the statistics will surely change. Most likely the pass rate will decline. Certainly we will then have a deeper appreciation of just how challenging the oral exam truly is.

Chapter 4

Getting Started

Priority of Study Topics

The oral exam can cover any topic related to Obstetrics, Gynecology and Women's Health. However, it is obviously impossible to review every topic. Perhaps the most common and costly mistake is failure to prioritize and focus your studying.

To prioritize, you must identify your personal strengths and weaknesses in specific topics. It is neither helpful nor realistic (yet typical of most compulsive physicians) to underestimate your strengths. Most candidates assume that they are weak, or at least in need of a review of all topics. The task of identifying and then prioritizing your knowledge base entails two critical steps.

The first step—and the most important while prioritizing—is to identify which topics are most likely to appear on the exam. Your case list is essentially an open book test. Take advantage of this and prepare for every topic on your list. You are accountable for every case list category, even if you didn't chose it for your case list. How to extrapolate which of these topics is most likely to appear on your exam is covered in Chapter 5 (The Case List). Effective in 2015, ABOG publishes a list of exam topics in the *ABOG Bulletin*. This list is similar to the case list categories, but with a bit more detail. Obviously you need to embrace each of these topics.

The second step is to identify your individual strengths and weaknesses in topics not yet covered above. Although there are as many different ways to tackle this problem as there are candidates, two techniques are popular.

The common features, however, are to be candid with your critique, to limit time and resources, and to revise your list periodically.

The first method is to take your Ob/Gyn textbooks and skim the table of contents for broad areas. For areas that you have identified as weak, skim further through the chapter for specific topics. The second method is to attend a review course approximately six months before your exam. Make three lists: top, medium, and low priority. As the lectures proceed, fill in the various topics on one of the respective lists.

Thus, the time spent in identifying your study priorities before you actually begin studying is well worth the time invested. You will markedly enhance your efficiency in the remaining study time. More importantly, however, you should start first the topics that are most likely to appear on your exam.

References

Certainly there are as many different references and resources as there are candidates. The most important variable in selecting your resources is to recognize that your goal is to *review* the topic. Failure to discipline yourself and to limit your review is the most common reason for running out of time; thus being unable to cover all of the topics on your priority study list.

The best safeguard is to select resources that are limited to a review of topics. Hence, the last reference to choose is a textbook, because its purpose is to provide an in-depth and exhaustive treatise of specific topics. Even so, the number of qualifying references is vast. Five sources consistently surface as being the most popular. The first three are ACOG publications that represent the standard of care and the last two are ABOG publications.

The first is *Precis*, an ACOG publication that is a concise summary of individual topics in Ob/Gyn. This reference is sweet and short and allows an excellent review in a time-efficient manner. The text is also written from a patient management perspective, which is the exact style for the oral board exam.

The second reference is the *PROLOG* series. PROLOG is an acronym for Personal Review of Learning on Obstetrics and Gynecology. These reviews consist of clinically oriented, multiple-choice questions with an editorial discussion of the answer. Although in a written exam format, they are an excellent source to judge your proficiency in individual topics. They can be used in the beginning to assist in identifying study topics, or at the end of a review to verify its thoroughness.

The most recommended resource is the ACOG *Compendium*. As its name implies, it is a compilation of clinical practice guidelines and consists of *Committee Opinions, Practice Bulletins, Policy Statements, Technology Assessments* and *Safety Checklists*.

The ACOG *Committee Opinions* are briefs about "clinical issues of an urgent or emergent nature or nonclinical topics such as policy, economics and social issues." They represent ACOG's stance on the hottest controversial issues confronting practitioners. Referencing these briefs during the exam substantiates a candidate's course of action, particularly if it deviates from the examiner's opinion.

Policy Statements are just that. They are the Colleges' position on key issues approved by the Executive Board. If you chose or practice the opposite stance, you definitely want to be able to defend why you are swimming against the current.

Technology Assessments describe specific technologies and their application. You should be familiar with these as the national standard of care, especially if you provide such services. The most common is ultrasound, a useful tool we use daily, whether performed by ourselves or our technician. It is so commonplace that we often take for granted the science behind the technology and quality control measures, both of which are hot test topics.

Practice Bulletins are evidence-based practice guidelines. They are the final answer on any issue since they are based on sound, peer-reviewed clinical research. They represent ACOG's and hence should also be your preferred method of diagnosis and management of a condition. They are your best source for a brief, to-the-point, clinical review of specific topics. Unquestionably, you should start your review of every topic with the corresponding *Practice Bulletin*; hopefully, you will also be able to end it there.

The *Safety Checklists* are the newest addition to the ACOG Compendium. They are analogous to the pilot preflight checklist, as they represent a checklist for commonly performed procedures. No doubt you will have some of these procedures on your case list, so it is paramount for you to literally check them off your list before you construct your case list or sit for your exam.

Even though you cannot start Maintenance of Certification (MOC) until after you pass your oral exam, MOC is affecting you now. Phase II of your MOC requires that you read and take an open book written examination on each of 45 articles each year. Guess who selects these articles? Right, ABOG. So you can bet these are topics that ABOG feels are important and they may likely carry over to your oral exam. I suggest you peruse the last two years of MOC articles. I don't feel it's necessary to read every article, but would recommend that you do so for those topics that overlap with your case list. Also, about a quarter of the MOC articles are Compendium references, so you definitely want to read those. Remember too, that your examiners also have to read these articles. The articles deadline is December, so they will be fresh in the examiner's mind for your fall oral exam.

Finally, the Foundation for Exxcellence in Women's Health, sponsored in part by ABOG, publishes *The Pearls of Exxcellence*, which is a monthly review of the most challenging topics on the oral exam. This is a sweet opportunity to get a rare insight into the exam topics and the desired focus.

The bottom line in selecting your references is to limit them. Choose resources that are restricted to a review of the topic. Textbooks are a last resort and should be used sparingly.

Review Courses

Let's first make sure we're on the same sheet of music by defining a review course. A review course is multiple days (at least five days duration) of didactic lectures covering a review of a wide spectrum of Ob/Gyn topics by multiple faculty members - both generalists and subspecialists. This is not to be confused with a tutorial service or a seminar that deceptively use the name review course.

Review courses are helpful for several reasons. They allow a pace and intensity of review that is difficult to match with independent study. Furthermore, they are an excellent gauge to prioritize study topics. Perhaps most important, however, is the "step-away" time that allows you to focus exclusively on studying. Several variables should be considered in selecting a course.

The reputation of a review course is a good place to start. Ask your colleagues what course(s) they attended. What was their reason for choosing that course? How long ago did they attend? Most importantly, would they attend it again and would they highly recommend it for you? This is a starting point, but you need to do your own due diligence to confirm that their recommendations match your needs.

The first consideration in choosing a review course is when to attend. Ideally, attend one just as you are peaking in your case list entry, which is typically late spring, such as April or May of the year of the exam. This timing has two distinct advantages: (1) it is the ideal time to prioritize your study topics and draft a study plan, and (2) it allows optimal incorporation of the strategy you learned in organizing the case list. As discussed before, half of the exam is based on the case list and the majority of failures are due to inadequate defense. Because the time from the end of the case list compilation (June 30) to the deadline for turning it in (August 1) is so tight, you must have a definitive plan to act quickly and efficiently to incorporate your strategy.

The next strategic time to take a review course is just before you start your intense studying, which should be about two or three months before the exam. You should choose a course that covers the topics that you have already identified as priorities. The course should also uncover overlooked topics, as well as topics that should be upgraded in priority.

The final opportune time is one or two weeks before the exam. The primary objective is to get into the mind-set for the test: to eat, drink, and sleep Ob/Gyn. The goal is simply to refresh previously studied topics. If you take the course at any earlier time (even a month before the exam), it is difficult to maintain the intensity and recall necessary for the test. This timing also affords the opportunity to "put it all together" by taking mock oral exams. Recall the steep slope of the learning curve. In learning a new task, you improve dramatically with each repetition. Since few candidates are experienced with the oral exam format, you will markedly improve your performance and your chance of passing by taking even only three mock orals. To walk into the oral exam cold, without having practiced specifically the oral exam format, is a foolish risk and potentially a waste of months of preparation.

In addition to timing, there are other factors that should be considered in selecting a review course. First and foremost, verify that the course is geared toward the oral exam. The name of the review course should state "BOARD review course," to distinguish it from a general review course. The timing of the course relative to the exam determines which features are offered. Certainly some lectures should be dedicated to exam strategy. Both didactic and private sessions on the case list should be offered. Verify that the course provides strategy for case list collection, construction and defense. Take advantage of private tutoring dedicated to your case list alone. Unquestionably, any course offered at least two to three months before your test date *must* offer mock oral exams. If it does not, look for one that does.

Expense is also a consideration. Review courses that offer a refund of the registration fee if you do not pass your exam cater specifically to those preparing for an exam, and not just to those looking for a general review.

However, make sure you read the fine print, as there are usually contingencies in order to receive your refund. The tuition or registration fee may be just the beginning. Look for hidden expenses that can put you over budget.

I recommend you consider the following expenses:

Registration fee:
>Do they offer a discount for
>>resident/fellow physicians in training?
>>
>>multiple registrants?
>>
>>early registration?
>>
>>armed forces members?
>>
>>returning registrant?
>>
>>package deals by combining products and services with course registration?
>
>Does it include meals and snacks?

Lodging:
>Does room rate include:
>>complimentary shuttle to/from airport?
>>
>>complimentary meals?
>>
>>complimentary internet access?
>
>What amenities are available:
>>in-room meal prep (kitchenette, microwave, fridge, etc.)?
>>
>>on-site or nearby restaurants?
>>
>>suite to keep studying separate from sleeping?
>>
>>fitness center?
>>
>>business center?
>>
>>swimming pool?
>>
>>Complimentary shuttle to nearby restaurants, shopping, etc.
>>
>>Is it safe? Can you go out for a walk or run?

To save money, consider:
>Sharing a room with a colleague to cut costs.
>
>Is it less expensive to stay at a different hotel and travel back and forth for lectures?

Bottom line, this is not a vacation conference. All day, and often the early evenings are spent in lectures or coaching sessions. Have your family accompany you only if they are keenly aware of your time commitments.

The length of the course is important. Realistically, how long can you stay focused? Most of us have not had to sit all day and listen to lectures since medical school. Although you will find this surprisingly enjoyable at first, your back and bladder are unconditioned and both your physical and intellectual stamina quickly falter within a few days. Emotionally, it's also a rude awakening to acknowledge just how much you have forgotten and what a monumental task it will take to get back up to speed. Furthermore, how much time can you afford to be away from your practice or residency? You must budget not just for the time needed for one course, but perhaps several courses, as well as for family (remember them?). Thus, I recommend you attend a 5-7 day course. Ideally, a course that overlaps with a weekend will minimize time away from your practice. Better yet, perhaps you can couple the review course with a 1 to 3 day tutorial course.

Finally, the faculty and the course agenda are the most variable features between the different courses. Because the goal is to review, it is not necessary—and actually may be a waste of time—to have noted academicians, since they have a tendency to include trivia and to focus on their latest research. The lecturers should focus on patient management issues consistent with the ACOG standards.

The course mailer or website should boast on the caliber of the faculty: not just on their expertise of the topic, but also on their experience as speakers. Be wary of courses that primarily use residents, fellows and junior faculty all from the same institution. Chances are they were assigned the topic and the data will be presented from that institution's perspective and not necessarily ACOG's. You should have the opportunity for hands-on time with the faculty for questions, and especially for mock oral exams and reviewing your case list. All the speakers must be clinicians. The oral exam is the ultimate clinical application of knowledge. If the review course faculty aren't in the OR, office, or labor and delivery daily, they have no business lecturing on the topic, nor giving you advice.

Furthermore, because it is impossible to cover every topic, each course will have a different agenda. Direct inquiry to the course administration should confirm their strategy. The right answer is that the topics were chosen based entirely on the likelihood of occurring on your exam.

Perhaps the most helpful tool for evaluating review courses is through the internet. With a few key strokes, you can conduct a quick and easy, yet thorough comparison of what is currently available. I would start with key search terms as "Ob/Gyn board review course" or "Ob/Gyn review course". A course's website, just like your case list, is an excellent thumbprint as to their philosophy. What is their attention to detail? Is the website current? Is it easy to navigate? Do the testimonials seem sincere and legitimate? Do you feel like you're being swindled? Is there a link designated for faculty or are they relegated to the miscellaneous tab? Can you register on-line? How quickly does the staff respond to your e-mail inquiries?

Many review courses are available on DVD and/or CD. You should not use these in lieu of attending a course. The substitute is never as good as the real thing. Attendance demands your complete captivity and allows for interaction with both faculty and colleagues. Unless the course was just recorded, the DVDs and CDs do not reflect the most recent updates, nor do they often contain evening sessions on exam tips and strategies. They are, however, an excellent resource to solidify and reinforce your studies. An excellent quality DVD should display the speaker and their slides simultaneously. The accompanying handouts are usually available on a CD or hard copy to follow along. The audio CDs are great reinforcement for those who have a commute and are also a nice accompaniment during exercise.

In summary, a review course (or courses) is a useful tool in your armamentarium of resources. The easiest and most helpful report card can be obtained by trusted colleagues who have attended courses previously. To benefit the most however, do your homework to determine which course(s) best fulfills your needs.

Tutorial Courses

A number of companies and review courses offer instruction and mentoring specific to the oral exam. These tutorial services, provided as an addendum to the review course, are separate and distinct from the course itself. They differ in that their focus is on strategy, whereas the review course focus is on content.

You should carefully evaluate what each tutorial service has to offer, just like you would for your review course. These tutorial services are either attended in person or virtually. In-house options are referred to as workshops, seminars, or camp; the on-line options are webinars. Ideally, the number of participants should be limited to no more than 20 to 30 people to ensure the opportunity for personal attention.

The tutorial course should cover topics on what to expect in the way of exam format and content, as well as tips on how to conduct yourself during the exam. It should outline the format of the exam so you know what to expect. Whereas the review course should review the topics, the tutorial course should discuss the necessary strategies. For example, a tutorial course will emphasize that shoulder dystocia is a hot topic and that you must know the maneuvers. The review course will *review* the topic shoulder dystocia, of which only one component is the various maneuvers.

The tutorial courses also coach you in preparation specifically for the oral exam. They usually offer assistance in the case list, including strategic construction and/or how to defend your case list. Finally, they should coach you in the technique of the oral exam. There should be some didactic lectures to educate you on the approach, but especially include the opportunity to practice your newfound skills with your cohorts and local/regional colleagues.

The icing on the cake however, is utilizing the course faculty. Although you can prepare capably on your own, typically you lack the same level of experience and expertise. The course faculty has two distinct attributes that you need. One is that they better reflect the ABOG examiner profile because they're specialists. If you're a generalist, you won't see your cases the same way the specialist will. Most importantly, the course faculty doesn't know you, so they can examine and evaluate you with unbiased objectivity. Bottom line, the course faculty can better simulate the exam environment and they are in a better position to give you specific tips for improvement to enhance your chances for passing your exam. The disadvantage is that they are an additional expense beyond the review course. However, in only a few sessions you can probably pick up your deficiencies to provide guidance to your resources back home so you can continue to practice and improve.

There are two ideal times to take a tutorial workshop in case list construction. The first is *before* you begin collecting your case list (e.g., late spring or early summer the year before your exam) to allow best utilization of tips on case list collection. In particular, this strategy avoids the frustration of choosing the wrong computer program for data entry. One of the most common responses to "What would you do differently?" is "I would have bailed out of the ABOG case list program." Unfortunately, by the time most candidates acknowledge their error, the time spent to reenter the data into a new program equals the time lost in continuing to struggle with the ABOG program.

Very few have the insight or are proactive enough to be this organized. Don't fret. Instead, take the workshop when you are about three quarters of the way into collecting your cases (e.g., late spring, such as April). By this time, you are familiar with the process and can be more attentive on the strategy, rather than the process. If you decide to bail out of the ABOG case list software, you will have plenty of time to switch systems and reenter your data. The bottom line is: get some professional guidance on how to artfully and strategically construct that case list *before* you submit it on August 1. You will be so glad you did, as it is so much easier to defend a well constructed case list. After August 1, that case list is set in stone.

The other ideal time to attend a workshop is one to two months before your exam. Now you know the exact topics on your case list. The focus is now how to *defend* it with competence and confidence. The tutorial course should prepare you both with didactics and hands-on practice via an oral exam.

The tutorial and review courses are not interchangeable; rather, they nicely complement each other. If you can only attend one or the other, then definitely attend the review course. However, the ultimate preparation would be to attend *both* a review course and a tutorial workshop.

It is imperative that you research and compare the different tutorial services. How long has the company been around? Who and how long have the faculty been teaching the workshop? Did the faculty mentor pass his exam the first time? Are all the mock oral examiners clinicians? What is their pass rate? Of course, the best recommendation is from a satisfied customer. A reputable course should readily offer you a list of references from past participants. The tutorial workshops allow you to put it all together. Here you find out what stuff you're made of. If you fail to perform satisfactorily, a good tutorial course will provide you with the tools needed to refine and polish your presentation.

Milestones

How did the pygmies eat the elephant? One bite at a time! I will give you a plan for *when* and *how big* your bites should be. It is based on the military tool of milestones, which are dates by which each specific task must be completed in order to accomplish the mission.

Developing the milestones chart is easy. Simply define the mission, determine the time required to complete the individual tasks, back plot the time, and voilà!—this is when you start. Saying it is one thing—doing it is quite another.

Chapter 4 • Getting Started

TABLE 1 Milestones for the Traditional Track

Time	Task
Fall (year preceding the exam)	Review course and/or Case list Construction Workshop
June (year preceding the exam)	Order previous years ABOG case list software
1 July–30 June	Case list collection
September/October	Order current ABOG case list software
February	Request application
February	Case List Construction Workshop, if not already
15 March	Application, fee, copy of medical license, and photographs due
16 March – 15 April	Late application plus late fee
16 April – 30 April	Late application plus additional late fee
30 April	No applications accepted after this date
1 May – 1 June	Case List Construction Workshop, if not already
15 May – 1 June	Send case list to critics for construction tips
April - June	Board review course and/or Case List Construction Workshop, if not already
30 June	Complete case list collection
July	Receive ABOG notification of admissibility to exam and month of exam
1–10 July	First case list draft completed
10 July	Send first draft to critics
10–28 July	Second case list draft completed
29 July	Medical records notarization Send case list and examination fee by certified mail
1 August	Case list deadline Examination fee deadline Send case list to critics for defense tips
4-14 August	Late examination fee, late case list fee
3-10 August	Break
14 August	No case lists or examination fees accepted
14–21 August	Collect resources Develop study plan
Mid August– September	Intense studying–focused on case list Break 1 day/week
September or October	Meet with critics to review case list defense strategy Board review course and/or Oral Exam Workshop

Pass Your Oral OB/GYN Board Exam!

Time	Task

October (if November exam)	Intense studying–focused on exam probability
	Mock oral exams
	    Generalist
	    Maternal/fetal medicine (MFM) specialist
	    Reproductive endocrinologist
	    Oncologist
	    Female Pelvic Medicine & Reconstructive Surgery (FPM)

October (if December exam)	Intense studying–focused on case list Break 1 day/week
November (if November exam)	Mock oral exams
November (if December exam)	Intense studying–focused on exam probability Board review course and/or Oral Exam Workshop Mock oral exams
November (if January exam)	Intense studying–focused on case list Break 1 day/week
December (if December exam)	Mock oral exams
December (if January exam)	Intense studying–focused on exam probability Board review course and/or Oral Exam Workshop Mock oral exams
January (if January exam)	Mock oral exams

TABLE 2 Milestones for the Fast Track

Time	Task
Last Monday June	Written Board Exam
1 July–30 June	Case list collection
June (year preceding the exam)	Order previous years ABOG case list software
1 July–30 June	Case list collection
1 August (year preceding the exam)	Notification of pass/fail on written exam
2 August	Automated application for oral exam and application fee due
12 September	No applications accepted after this date
September/October	Order current ABOG case list software
1 October	Notification if accepted into accelerated process
15 May – 1 June	Send case list to critics for construction tips
April - June	Board review course and/or Case List Construction Workshop, if not already
30 June	Complete case list collection
July	Receive ABOG notification of admissibility to exam and month of exam

Chapter 4 • Getting Started

Time	Task
1–10 July	First case list draft completed
10 July	Send first draft to critics
10–28 July	Second case list draft completed
29 July	Medical records notarization Send case list and examination fee by certified mail
1 August	Case list deadline Examination fee deadline Send case list to critics for defense tips
4-14 August	Late examination fee, late case list fee
3-10 August	Break
14 August	No case lists or examination fees accepted
14–21 August	Collect resources Develop study plan
Mid August– September	Intense studying–focused on case list Break 1 day/week
September or October	Meet with critics to review case list defense strategy Board review course and/or Oral Exam Workshop

October (if November exam)	Intense studying–focused on exam probability
	Mock oral exams
	    Generalist
	    Maternal/fetal medicine (MFM) specialist
	    Reproductive endocrinologist
	    Oncologist
	    Female Pelvic Medicine & Reconstructive Surgery (FPM)

October (if December exam)	Intense studying–focused on case list Break 1 day/week
November (if November exam)	Mock oral exams
November (if December exam)	Intense studying–focused on exam probability Board review course and/or Oral Exam Workshop Mock oral exams
November (if January exam)	Intense studying–focused on case list Break 1 day/week
December (if December exam)	Mock oral exams
December (if January exam)	Intense studying–focused on exam probability Board review course and/or Oral Exam Workshop Mock oral exams
January (if January exam)	Mock oral exams

TABLE 3 Milestones for the Fast Track for Fellows

Time	Task
Last Monday in June	Written Board Exam for incoming fellows
Last Monday June	Written Board Exam for incoming fellows
1 July of 1st, 2nd, 3rd, or 4th fellowship year	Begin case list collection
June (year preceding the exam)	Order previous years ABOG case list software
1 August (year preceding the exam)	Notification of pass/fail on written exam
2 August	Automated application for oral exam and application fee due
12 September	No applications accepted after this date
September/October	Order current ABOG case list software
1 October	Notification if accepted into accelerated process
15 May – 1 June	Send case list to critics for construction tips
April - June	Board review course and/or Case List Construction Workshop, if not already
30 June	Complete case list collection
July	Receive ABOG notification of admissibility to exam and month of exam
1–10 July	First case list draft completed
10 July	Send first draft to critics
10–28 July	Second case list draft completed
29 July	Medical records notarization Send case list and examination fee by certified mail
1 August	Case list deadline Examination fee deadline Send case list to critics for defense tips
4-14 August	Late examination fee, late case list fee
3-10 August	Break
14 August	No case lists or examination fees accepted
14–21 August	Collect resources Develop study plan
Mid August– September	Intense studying–focused on case list Break 1 day/week
September or October	Meet with critics to review case list defense strategy Board review course and/or Oral Exam Workshop

October (if November exam)	Intense studying–focused on exam probability
	Mock oral exams
	  Generalist
	  Maternal/fetal medicine (MFM) specialist
	  Reproductive endocrinologist
	  Oncologist
	  Female Pelvic Medicine & Reconstructive Surgery (FPM)

Time	Task
October (if December exam)	Intense studying–focused on case list Break 1 day/week
November (if November exam)	Mock oral exams
November (if December exam)	Intense studying–focused on exam probability Board review course and/or Oral Exam Workshop Mock oral exams
November (if January exam)	Intense studying–focused on case list Break 1 day/week
December (if December exam)	Mock oral exams
December (if January exam)	Intense studying–focused on exam probability Board review course and/or Oral Exam Workshop Mock oral exams
January (if January exam)	Mock oral exams

Tables 1, 2 and 3 summarize the milestones for traditional and fast tracks, respectively. The estimate of the time required for each step will vary with each person. Candid, realistic soul-searching must be invested to analyze how best to modify the milestones for you. Periodically review the timetable and adjust it accordingly to accomplish the end goal.

The secret for success with the milestone system is timing. Timing is the art of synchronizing events to result in the optimal outcome: in other words…when all the pieces of the puzzle fall into place. Timing is critical in three areas: the case list organization, peer review and the study plan.

Because the time from the end of the case list data collection (June 30) to the deadline for turning it in (August 1) is so tight, you must have a definite plan to act quickly and incorporate your strategy. I have yet to meet a candidate who was pleased with the original draft. As a matter of fact, one of the most common regrets of previous candidates is not allowing enough time to edit. Ideally, you were able to take advantage of a case list construction workshop earlier and already have a plan to implement your strategy and are readily familiar with the software to quickly enter edits. The four weeks allotted for organization of the case list allows time for only one rewrite.

The first draft of the completed case list should be accomplished by mid-July. To meet this deadline, the recommendations from your reviewers must be received no later than July 1. Obviously, you must give them their respective sections in time to accommodate their schedule.

With approximately four weeks remaining, most candidates have time for only one rewrite. Again, you are at the mercy of your reviewer's schedule to incorporate the second set of recommendations. Apologetically make clear the deadline you need for them to meet to allow you time to incorporate their suggestions. To avoid running out of time, edit as soon as each case is ready, rather than when the entire case list is done.

Since half the exam is based on defending your case list, the initial time spent on strategic organization will be much appreciated when you plan your defense. This is your only chance to influence the examiner's first impression, since he or she receives the case list before the first handshake on the day of the exam. This is the first time that many candidates have begun to think seriously about preparing for the exam; clearly those who charge into battle on July 1 have the edge.

The second critical milestone category is peer review. Critique of your case list, as well as mock oral exams, is invaluable. Reviewers will see the obvious that you outright missed. The first opportunity for case list review is when your compilation is nearing the end. Send the obstetrics section to your referring maternal-fetal medicine specialist and/or a local generalist, the gynecologic section to your oncologist, female pelvic medicine, and/or generalist, and the office practice section to your reproductive endocrinologist or generalist. The specialist more than likely will reflect the profile of the examiner, but the local generalist will be more familiar with your mode of practice. For a professional opinion, seek out one of the review courses or tutorial courses that has a seasoned faculty, experienced in reviewing case lists, that will trouble shoot your case list and offer savvy tips on construction.

Allow ample time for review, but also be up front about your deadline. Send the first batch in May or June and set a due date of July 1. Send the next draft back to the reviewer by mid-July with a due date in the third week of July. The purpose of this peer review from May through July is to make recommendations for the strategic organization and construction of the case list. Send the masterpiece back in August and/or September. The goal then is to help plan its defense. You may again want a pair of professional eyes to identify expected questions, and especially ideal answers, for your exam.

The ultimate test of your depth and breadth of knowledge and ability to convey it is the mock oral exam. Because most of us are unfamiliar with, and hence intimidated by its format, there is a natural tendency to procrastinate or worse yet, to avoid this valuable study tool. Most physicians are stereotypically their own worst critics. They underestimate their abilities and delay a mock oral to bone up even more and to avoid the embarrassing acknowledgment that they don't know everything. This tactic is self-defeating because your peers already know that you can't possibly know it all.

I recommend a planning session in September for the case list defense strategy with each of the colleagues to whom you sent the segments for case list organization tips. Most valuable of all is to schedule a mock oral exam with each colleague the month before your exam. The final test is a mock oral exam with a peer(s) who is unfamiliar to you, such as the review or tutorial course faculty member. Again, this may be better left to the professionals whose recommendations are based on years of feedback of their tried and true tips.

After the case list is set in stone, the final major milestone is to determine *what* you need to study and *when*. The *what* process is outlined in Chapter 8 (Studying for the Exam). Recall that study topics are prioritized by exam probability. The prioritizing of these topics is based on your comfort with your knowledge base of each topic.

Determining *when*, or more specifically how long to devote to each study topic, is an art learned only through experience. It is gained only upon realizing that studying for the oral boards is completely different from studying for the written boards. To study for the orals in the same manner as for the written boards is a waste of precious time. A written exam by nature is restricted to individual questions within a specific topic. The written exam ends with the answer to the question, whereas the oral exam starts with the answer to the question. The oral exam is an evaluation of your collective understanding of the topic and your ability to apply that knowledge to patient management. Thus, studying for the oral exam should be limited to a comprehensive, clinically oriented review—not an exhaustive, in-depth understanding laden with textbook facts.

Incredible discipline is required to restrict your study to a review. Tackling the first few topics is all that is necessary to learn the new focus and to gain an appreciation of the time required to cover a topic. After you get the hang of it, go back and revise your original study timetable accordingly.

In conclusion, timing is everything. The oral exam is clearly an example of the proverb "forewarned is forearmed". Undoubtedly, anyone who has passed the written board exam is academically capable of passing their oral boards. But those who methodically and diligently stick to their plan will accomplish this feat much more easily

Chapter 5
The Case List

Significance of the Exam

The ABOG *Bulletin* states that half of your exam is defending your case list. The case list is a far more accurate assessment of your mode of practice than a mere three hours of testing. It is the culmination of applying book knowledge to clinical practice for a full year. Thus, in my opinion, the most important variable of all exam components is the case list.

The examiners receive your case list at least the day before your exam. Certainly the degree of scrutiny varies with each examiner and the number of case lists he receives. Nevertheless, the examiner meets your case list before he meets you. Undoubtedly, he will form a first impression of you based exclusively on your case list.

I have reviewed many case lists. Outright failures, although rare, are obvious. On the other hand, there are no guaranteed passes based on the case list alone. The other test components (e.g. structured cases) and especially your finesse with the oral exam format, greatly influence the outcome. However, as long as you do not outright flunk the other exam components, you will surely pass the exam if you have satisfactorily defended your case list.

Thus, sound performance on the oral exam and a solid case list defense are a sure bet for passing. An unsound case list, regardless of a stellar performance on the exam, will most likely result in failure. An unsound case list and a weak performance on the exam are guaranteed to result in failure.

Criteria for Admission to the Exam

The case list is a compilation of office and hospital patients for whom you personally provided care during the 12 months preceding June 30 of the year of your exam. This implies that you, not your partner or residents, personally controlled the medical and/or surgical management of each patient listed. You cannot reuse any case/case list from a previous examination. If you are a generalist, you must submit a case list in all three areas. If your practice is limited to obstetrics *or* gynecology, you must submit a case list in your area of specialty and a minimum of 20 patients selected from your chief year in the off area. Regardless, you will be examined in *all three areas*: obstetrics, gynecology, and office practice.

All candidates must have an office and a hospital practice. The case list must include 40 office practice patients *and* a minimum of 20 hospitalized and/or ambulatory gynecologic *and* 20 hospitalized obstetric patients with significant problems.

If the minimum 20 obstetrical and 20 gynecological hospital-based patients cannot be obtained in the defined one-year period, you have two options. You can submit an additional *complete* six month case list of the patients managed immediately prior to the 12-month period, namely January 1 to June 30. The other option is to submit patients from your chief year of residency to complete the list of 20 gynecological and/or 20 obstetrical cases. You cannot submit a case list comprised solely of cases from your chief year. Thus, you will then submit two lists with a minimum of 20 hospitalized patients for 12 months duration and one of 6 months duration, and/or a case list from your chief year.

Case lists for subspecialists must meet the same criteria discussed above for those practitioners with a limited practice. In other words, your case list must contain obstetrical and gynecological cases either from your practice and/or from your fellowship or chief residency. Unlike the generalists however, your minimum of 20 cases on your off-specialty list can be comprised entirely from your chief residency cases.

Until 2014, subspecialty fellows were not allowed to take their general oral boards earlier than the second year and only once during their fellowship. Now, however, you can take your general oral boards anytime in your fellowship. You can also take your subspecialty written boards anytime in your fellowship, assuming that you've passed your primary written board exam. However, you cannot sit for your subspecialty oral boards until you pass your general oral boards.

If your chief list is more than five years since residency, in 2013 and 2014 ABOG assigned you a list. However in 2015, the *Bulletin* cited that if you cannot meet the minimum number in one area after using an 18 month list, nor the residency cases, you must contact ABOG citing the reasons why. A committee will then review your situation and decide what to do.

If this is as clear as mud, I suggest you check with the ABOG *Bulletin* or write ABOG for clarification. Actually it's a good idea to cross reference to the *Bulletin* regardless, in order to catch any new changes. I want to emphasize that ALL candidates will be tested in ALL THREE areas: obstetrics, gynecology, and office practice.

Collection of the Case List

No other phase of preparation for the exam requires as much discipline as the collection of your case list. Since it is a year-long compilation, there is a tendency to procrastinate. Not surprisingly, however, procrastination creates a domino effect—last-minute scrambling and haste that truly makes waste. Precious details are best recalled when fresh.

There are three sections to the case list: obstetrics, gynecology, and office practice. ABOG provides the forms with the specific format for recording each section (see Appendix D). Every gynecologic surgery and hospitalized obstetric patient must be logged, whereas only 40 patients from the office practice categories are necessary.

Recall from Chapter 2 (The Application Process) that you cannot formally request an application until February of the year of your exam. Yet the time frame for the case list started way back on July 1. To delay until February results in a dangerous, self-perpetuating backlog because ongoing data continue to accrue.

To avoid always being behind the eight ball, I recommend that you obtain the preceding year's forms by July 1. The only risk is that the form format may change (but it hasn't in years), necessitating reentry of data. The benefit of timely data collection far outweighs the unlikely risk of having to transfer data to updated forms.

How often you should update your case list is highly variable. Feedback from previous candidates reveals the average time is weekly. The ideal time, in my opinion, is after every patient, when recall is at its peak. The least frequent update, without risk for significantly compromising recall, is bimonthly.

The method of recording the data depends on individual preference. In any case, the initial log should be readily transportable, either by paper or web-/cloud-based. Enter the case immediately after every delivery or surgery.

The office practice case list collection is no less challenging, even though it is only 40 patients. Although it is not necessary to begin collecting these patients on July 1, there is a tendency to procrastinate and all of a sudden be behind. Additionally, you must put some thought into which of the 36 categories you want to represent; whereas you don't have a choice on the obstetrics or gynecology list. Keep the list of all categories on your desk. Add the names of the representative patients no later than January.

Common office practice categories, such as menopause, vaginitis and preventive care, will fill up quickly. Since a maximum of two patients can be listed in each category, it is not necessary to collect more than four patients. Less common categories, such as pediatric gynecology and sexual assault, may take months, if possible at all, to find. Collection of patients in rare categories is obviously most compromised by procrastination. There are a total of 41 categories. The more categories you can use, the better this will reflect your depth and breadth of clinical acumen. It's uncommon to use more than 30 categories, and I've yet to see a case list use all 40 unique categories.

The first rough draft needs to be edited and entered in accordance with the ABOG requirements. You may either submit the data to your transcriptionist or enter it yourself. There are pros and cons for each option. Do not waste time if you are unfamiliar or unskilled with either. Be efficient with revisions; make them purposeful and strategic. Knowing what to edit is not usually obvious until the entire case list is entered. Since compilation ends June 30 and the case list is due August 1, little time remains for more than two major revisions.

You can save time by having someone else enter your data on the ABOG forms. This option allows you to "step away" from that section and tackle the revisions later. You must, however, make your intent crystal-clear to avoid losing time in correcting miscommunications. The most obvious disadvantage is that you are dependent on someone else's schedule. Make it clear that the clock is ticking, and give specific deadlines. Remember also that procrastination on your part does not justify an emergency on theirs.

You can avoid these hassles by entering the data yourself. ABOG offers a computer software program, and because it is endorsed by ABOG, many candidates erroneously assume that it is the only acceptable program. This is not true. Any program may be used as long as it complies with the specific ABOG format requirements.

The ABOG program has some bugs, generates frustration and wastes time. Feedback from candidates who have tried both the ABOG program and one of their own design is hands down in favor of their own. Tips on how to do so (and on how to use the ABOG program) are in Appendix D. Choose the program that seems to you the easiest and most adaptable to editing.

Finally, you must personally tally your summary sheets by hand. The ABOG program and often even customized programs, do not count correctly. I recommend you have several checks and balances to make sure that your tally is accurate. Keep a log of every hospitalized obstetric and gynecologic patient. In addition, create a log based on each of the categories listed in the summary sheet. Include a description of each category if the categories are ambiguous. List the corresponding patient's name, date, and diagnosis or procedure for quick cross-reference. Most importantly, check your numbers—and check them twice.

Initial Draft: Case-by-Case Entry

The case list will make you or break you. Thus, you should painstakingly plan its organization and your defense. For each patient, draft a narrative summary of the patient management issues as if you were presenting her at morning report or teaching rounds. This clinical summary is the stepping stone from which you will later extract the pertinent data to complete the ABOG forms. Now let's discuss each of the three sections.

List of Obstetric Patients

List *separately* each patient with a complication or abnormality, along with medical and surgical interventions during pregnancy, labor, delivery and the puerperium. Although the final copy will list only complicated patients, I recommend you draft a clinical narrative for every delivery. Sometimes it is not obvious into which category a patient falls until later review.

You will simply list the total **number** of normal, uncomplicated obstetrical patients on the summary sheet. You will not list these patients individually on your case list like you will for the complicated ones. ABOG defines a normal uncomplicated patient by the following criteria:

A. Pregnancy, labor, delivery and the puerperium were uncomplicated, labor began spontaneously between the 39th and 41st week of gestation
B. The membranes ruptured or were ruptured after labor began
C. Presentation was vertex, position occiput anterior, left or right occiput anterior and labor was less than 24 hours in duration
D. Delivery was spontaneous or by outlet forceps with or without episiotomy, from an anterior position
E. The infant had a five-minute Apgar score of 6 or more, weighed between 2500 and 4500 grams, and was healthy
F. Uncomplicated delivery of the placenta and blood loss less than 500 ml.

All deliveries not fulfilling these criteria must be listed separately. The total number of deliveries (> 500 grams), both complicated and uncomplicated, are tallied at the end of the obstetric list and also on the summary sheet.

A minimum of 20 patients is required on the obstetrics list from the categories listed below. Although you must list *all* complicated patients, you cannot *apply* more than *two* patients from each category to meet the minimum requirement of 20 patients. For example, if you list four breech presentations in the "Breech and other Fetal Malpresentations" category, you must report all four in the "Total Cases" column of the summary sheet, but only two of the four will be counted or applied as meeting the minimum requirement of 20 cases. Don't misinterpret the total cases column with the need to include all the cases on your list that overlap with that category. In other words, if you have a total of six breeches on your list, but two of them were included in other categories, such as cord problems or hypertensive disorders, the total cases in the breech column is still four and the total in the applied is still no more than two. Check the ABOG Bulletin for the most up-to-date list of categories.

Obstetrical Categories
1. Abnormal fetal growth
2. Autoimmune disorders of pregnancy
3. Breech and other fetal malpresentations
4. Cardiovascular and/or pulmonary diseases complicating pregnancy
5. Cesarean hysterectomy
6. Complications of cesarean delivery

7. Complications of OB anesthesia
8. Cord problems
9. Dystocia
10. Fetal heart rate abnormalities
11. Hematologic diseases and/or endocrine diseases complicating pregnancy
12. Hypertensive disorders of pregnancy (chronic hypertension, preeclampsia, eclampsia)
13. Induction and/or augmentation of labor
14. Infectious diseases
15. Intrapartum or intra-amniotic infection (amnionitis, chorioamnionitis)
16. Labor abnormalities
17. Multifetal pregnancies
18. Obstetrical vaginal lacerations (3rd and 4th degree lacerations)
19. Obstetrical hemorrhage
20. Operative vaginal delivery (vacuum, forceps)
21. Placental abnormalities
22. Post-term pregnancy
23. Preconception evaluation, prenatal and genetic diagnoses
24. Pregnancies complicated by human immunodeficiency virus (HIV) infection
25. Pregnancies and coexisting malignancies
26. Premature rupture of membranes at term (PROM)
27. Preterm delivery
28. Preterm premature rupture of membranes (PPROM)
29. Pregnancies complicated by fetal anomalies
30. Primary Cesarean delivery
31. Psychiatric diseases complicating pregnancy
32. Puerperal infection
33. Renal diseases and/or neurologic diseases complicating pregnancy
34. Repeat Cesarean delivery

35. Second-trimester spontaneous abortion
36. Third-trimester fetal loss
37. Thrombotic complications
38. Trauma in pregnancy
39. Ultrasonography
40. Vaginal birth after cesarean delivery (VBAC)
41. Vaginal or perineal hematoma
42. Uncategorized

Whereas each complicated obstetric patient is listed, only the total number of normal, uncomplicated obstetric patients is tallied on the summary sheet. To ensure listing only appropriate patients, initially complete the ABOG form for ALL deliveries. You can later delete the uncomplicated patients after you are certain they are indeed a normal delivery.

The summary sheet should be hand tallied. Record ALL the patients that you managed in each category in the "Total Cases" column. This reflects your depth of experience in each category. Recall however, that you can only apply two patients from each category to count toward your mandatory minimum of 20 patients. These are recorded on the "Total Applied" column. The sum of the total applied is placed in the "Total Cases" column and must be 20 or more. The total number of deliveries will be the sum of the "Total Cases" and "Total Uncomplicated Spontaneous Deliveries" categories.

"OB Ultrasounds and Color Doppler Examinations" is the number of ultrasounds performed by *you* upon *hospitalized* obstetrical patients. Note again—this is the number that you personally performed, not those that you ordered and were performed by a technician or radiologist.

The Cesarean Delivery (CD) categories on the summary sheet do not necessarily represent your Cesarean delivery rate. Although a patient may have indeed had a CD, she may be applied in a different category. For example, if you performed a CD for a patient with a breech presentation, you may list her in either the "Breech and other Fetal Malpresentations" or "Cesarean Delivery" category, but not both. Even though the summary sheet no longer has a category for overall number of CDs, you must know your primary, repeat and total CD rate. If you are asked, you will have a ready answer, as in the middle of your exam is surely not a good time to get your calculator out.

The number of other obstetrical considerations is the final category of the summary sheet. This consists of "Apgars ≤5, infants <2500grams, and Perinatal Deaths". Each of these categories is also a separate heading in the columns of the Obstetric list. Thus, it is easy for the examiner to cross reference these from the summary sheet to the case list by quickly searching out the out-layers in their respective columns.

ABOG's only guidance on what to include on the entry sheet is the column headings. Don't misinterpret the antepartum complications column as only labor issues. This column should also include complications that occurred throughout the prenatal course. Laborists often struggle with how much, if any, of the antepartum issues to list if they didn't participate in the patient's care antenatally. Although you weren't involved in the decision making, you do have knowledge of these antenatal issues if you took a complete history. The disadvantage of listing only labor issues is the examiner has a free rein to come up with any hypothetical prenatal topic of his choice. Common sense should prevail; challenges in patient care don't start with the first contraction, but rather from the time of conception. You can always add a qualifier such as "antenatal care per another provider".

Although the content of the columns varies in subjectivity, understand what each column represents. Column confusion is the *most common mistake* in constructing the obstetric case list. The columns most often confused are *Complications of Antepartum, Complications of Delivery or Postpartum*, and *Operative Procedures and/or Treatment*. Include only the information that applies to that specific column. The confusion is due to differing interpretations in distinguishing antepartum from delivery. When does antepartum end and delivery begin?

Unfortunately, the customary division of labor into three stages does not fully clarify the debate. The first stage of labor begins with the onset of uterine contractions sufficient to efface the cervix and ends with complete cervical dilatation. The second stage of labor begins with complete cervical dilatation and ends with the expulsion of the infant. The third stage of labor is the separation and expulsion of the placenta.

Thus the *Antepartum* column clearly includes complications of pregnancy and the first stage of labor. Likewise, the *Delivery or Postpartum* column includes any complications of the third stage of labor and up to 6 weeks postpartum. In which column do stage II complications belong? Is delivery all of stage II, including pushing? Or is delivery purely the actual extraction or expulsion of the fetus? You can make an argument to include stage II complications in either the *Antepartum* or the *Delivery or Postpartum* column. Whichever you choose, be consistent throughout your case list.

I recommend that any complications up to and including complete cervical dilatation be listed in the *Antepartum* column. This includes disorders of protracted dilatation and arrest of dilatation. Any complication thereafter —namely, arrest of descent, instrumented deliveries and shoulder dystocia— can be listed in either the *Antepartum* or *Delivery or Postpartum* column.

Table 5.11 summarizes recommended listings for common complications, as well as possible treatment options.

TABLE 5.11 Recommended Listings and Treatment Options for Common Complications

Complication	Antepartum	Delivery or Postpartum	Operative Procedure and/or Treatment
Protracted labor	X		Pitocin augmentation
Arrest of dilatation	X		Pitocin augmentation and/or CD
Arrest of descent	X	X	Vacuum/forceps or CD
Cephalopelvic disproportion	X	X	Cesarean delivery
Shoulder dystocia		X	List of maneuvers optional
Retained placenta		X	Manual extraction
Uterine atony		X	Uterotonic agent

Example 1 (page 78) shows how the complications of protracted labor and Category II FHR were listed in the wrong column. They should be listed in the *Complications of Antepartum* column, not in the *Complications of Delivery and Postpartum* column. I hope to convince you later in the chapter, in the "Strategic Organization of the Case List" section, that the selection of the column especially reflects your logical and chronological thought process of patient management.

Be reasonable in your interpretation of a complication. I interpret a complication as any event or issue that *significantly* influences your management. You do not want to bog down your case list with copious insignificant data. For example, I would not list a patient if the only issue in an otherwise uncomplicated pregnancy, labor and delivery was advanced maternal age. On the other hand, if the patient became preeclamptic or carried a fetus with a trisomy, advanced maternal age might be listed as a complication (although you have to list the patient's age in any case). Similarly, I would not list teenage pregnancy, smoker, Rh negative, etc., unless these issues significantly complicated her care.

A simple rule of thumb is to decide whether you would present the patient in your morning report or changeover. If the answer is yes, list her; otherwise, count her as normal and uncomplicated.

How you word a problem greatly influences its interpretation and defense. If it's best to call a rose a rose, then do so. This is especially true if you have only one representative case. In other words, if you have only one gestational diabetic, then be specific in her management in the procedures &/or treatment column. The *Bulletin* makes a point to state that the examiner should have enough information to follow your work up and management. So back to Example 1: The candidate wisely specified her type of GDM as a White's A-1. However, if she were his only GDM patient, he fell short of clarifying her management as simply "routine diabetic care". He should have included "Nutritional Counseling, Glucose Surveillance, Growth Ultrasounds, Biweekly NSTs", so the examiner knows how he manages GDM. However, it's overkill if you keep repeating such specific detail for like patients. So, per Example 1, if the candidate had several GDM-A1s on his case list, then "routine diabetic care" would be appropriate. A good rule of thumb is: if it's the only topic or if you have a number of representative cases of the same topic, be specific with the first case and repeat the detail on like patients every couple of pages, otherwise be generic.

If you chose to be generic however, you must have a sprinkling of the specifics, so the examiner can deduce what you mean by routine care. For the most part, it's clear as to how you manage diabetics. IF he wants further details, he can ask you. However, if you worded the treatment for all your patients with the same problem generically, it is unknown as to how you manage such patients. This is risky, for if the examiner does not get time to validate the specifics, he is forced to assume you don't know. Like the medical chart, if it's not documented, it didn't happen. Recall also that the subspecialist examiner's definition of "routine" may be profoundly different than yours as a generalist.

The columns that dictate objective data are straightforward: *Patient #, Hospital #, Age, Gravida, Days in Hospital, Perinatal Death, Newborn Weight,* and *Apgar*. Initially, include the patient's name to aid in recall of the case. But absolutely, your final copy must de-identify her in order to be compliant with the Health Insurance Portability and Accounting Act of 1996 (HIPAA).

In 2008, and for several years thereafter, ABOG allowed you to have the patient's initials on the copy of the case list that you intended to use for the exam. However, the last several years, they dropped this verbiage from the *Bulletin*, but included it in your case list acceptance letter. I recommend you embrace that final de-identified list that you submitted, and do not to rely on initials, should they subsequently preclude allowing initials.

The "#" refers to the sequential ordering for all patients from all hospitals, so every patient will have a unique number. This is what the examiner refers to when he says, "Tell me about patient # __". The *hospital* # refers to the sequential ordering of hospitals being reported from. For example, if you admit patients to two hospitals, then they will be Hospital A and B, respectively. The *patient* # refers to the sequential ordering of patients reported from a given hospital. So let's say you deliver two patients from two different hospitals. The first is #1, and her *hospital* # is "A", so her *patient* # is "A-1". Whereas the second patient is #2, and her *hospital* # is "B", so her *patient* # is "B-1".

Parity means just that; do not enumerate further with abortions, preterm delivery, living offspring or ectopic pregnancies. List the *Gestational Age* at admission and round off in whole numbers, not fractions (e.g., 41 weeks, not 41 2/7 or 41+).

The *days in the hospital* are the number of days—not the dates. The newborn's *weight* is reported in grams.

Don't forget to note at the top of each case list page whether the source of each case was from *Post Residency Cases, Senior Residency Cases* or *Fellowship Cases*. Traditionally, it was not as obvious that a case list belonged to a subspecialist unless there were exactly 20 patients. However, now it's flashing in marquee lights at the top of each page. I doubt this allows for any mercy for the candidate defending his non-specialty or on the other hand, to be more scrutinized in the specialty area. The criteria for pass/fail should be the same for all. Note however, that the examiners tend to be subspecialists.

Be precise in terminology, especially for dysfunction of labor. At a minimum, use the appropriate Friedman terminology to justify augmentation of labor and cesarean deliveries. Certainly the duration threshold originally proposed for labor dysfunction, especially in the setting of an epidural, has come under fire recently. The key is to avoid the diagnosis "failure to progress" because it is vague and does not convey an understanding of the pathophysiology of labor. Make sure that your procedure and treatment are substantiated by the indicating complication.

I remind you again, it is imperative that you submit a de-identified case list to ABOG. Failure to do so will result in your case list being summarily rejected. Not only do you not get to Pass Go, but you also do not collect $200. You do, however, get to collect a whole new case list for next year!

Let's tie together all of the above suggestions for initial case entry by an example.

Clinical Summary

Karen Burke is a 34-year-old 2G/0P/1Ab at 38 weeks EGA. Karen had chronic hypertension that had not required medication. As the pregnancy progressed, she developed superimposed pre-eclampsia and required Aldomet.

At her 38-week office visit, her blood pressure was 160/110, a five pound weight gain since last week, and 2+ protein. She also complained of a severe headache.

She is sent to Labor & Delivery. Her cervix is unripe with a Bishop score of 3; therefore, she first undergoes successful cervical ripening with misoprostol. Pitocin induction is initiated, and she progresses to active labor but fails to dilate beyond 5 cm after two hours. An intrauterine pressure catheter is placed and demonstrates adequate Monte Video units, thereby confirming arrest of the active phase of labor. She is delivered by primary cesarean section. The infant weighs 3435 grams and has Apgar scores of 9 and 10.

Initial ABOG Form Entry

Start a binder for each of the three sections, Obstetrics, Gynecology, and Office Practice. Let's start with Obstetrics. For each OB patient, insert the clinical summary and the first draft of the ABOG form (see Example 2 on page 78). Ideally, include a copy of her prenatal record and the delivery note. If the patient was particularly complicated, you can supplement further with pertinent copies of other medical records, such as consults, laboratory, ultrasound reports, etc. Later you will add supporting resources and case list edits.

Begin a hand log of the statistics required on the Summary Sheet. Do not rely on the computer for accuracy. Many programs are fraught with inaccurate tallying.

OK, at this point at least we're out of the starting block. Don't get hung up on the logistics and the nitty gritty detail. That will come later. As a matter of fact, forget the doggone software if it's confusing and precluding you from starting. Remember the 'ole paper and pen?

Just use your common sense to enter the cases on the case list form. I promise you, once you get the hang of it, and it won't take long, you'll be primed to move to the next step. Remember long ago when you were an intern in labor and delivery? The first step was just learning how to do a cervical check. This is no different.

List of Gynecologic Patients

All patients who underwent a gynecologic surgical procedure outside the office setting and all nonsurgical admissions are listed. The total number of ultrasounds that you personally performed on hospitalized gynecologic patients must also be included, as well as the number of hospital stays >7 days.

A minimum of 20 gynecologic patients is required. Although you enter the total number of procedures performed in the "Total Cases" column, you may only count two patients from each of the categories listed below. Make sure to check the ABOG Bulletin for the most up-to-date list of categories.

Gynecological Categories

1. Abdominal Hysterectomy (total, subtotal, laparoscopic, robotic)
2. Abnormal Uterine Bleeding
3. Adnexal Problems excluding Ectopic Pregnancy and Pelvic Inflammatory Disease
4. Congenital Abnormalities of the Reproductive Tract
5. Diagnostic Laparoscopy
6. D&C
7. Ectopic Pregnancy (surgical management)
8. Emergency care
9. Endometriosis & Adenomyosis (surgical management)
10. Gestational trophoblastic disease
11. Incomplete, septic, complete and other abortion
12. Intraoperative complications (blood loss, hemorrhage, bowel injury, urinary tract injury)
13. Invasive Carcinoma
14. Laparotomy
15. Management of rectovaginal or urinary tract fistula
16. Operative Hysteroscopy
17. Operative Laparoscopy (other than Tubal Sterilization and Hysterectomy)
18. Operative Management of Pelvic Pain

19. Pelvic Inflammatory Disease
20. Postoperative Complications (hemorrhage, wound, urinary tract, GI, Pain, thrombotic, embolic, neurologic, fever, etc)
21. Preoperative Evaluation of Coexisting Conditions (respiratory, cardiac, metabolic diseases)
22. Repair of pelvic floor defects (prolapse)
23. Surgical management of VIN, CIN, and VAIN
24. Tubal Sterilization
25. Urinary and Fecal Incontinence (Operative Management)
26. Uterine Myomas
27. Vaginal Hysterectomy (including Laparoscopically Assisted)
28. Uncategorized

The "Total Applied" column in the Gynecologic Summary sheet cannot have more than two and the "Total Cases" of "Total Applied" must be at least 20. The "Total Cases" reflects how busy you are. The examiner can quickly determine a profile of the type of surgeon you are by simply perusing the number of cases of each category. The number of hospital stays that exceed seven days is an indicator of a complication, because who stays more than one or two days anymore? The examiner can quickly search the column within your case list and confirm his hunches.

As noted for the obstetrics list, understand what each column in the gynecologic form represents and complete each accordingly. The *preoperative or admission diagnosis* typically supports the treatment. The preoperative diagnosis should include pertinent nonsurgical, as well as conservative surgical therapy. For example, the pre-operative diagnosis of heavy menstrual bleeding (HMB) could be further qualified by lack of response to hormonal therapy or a D&C.

As discussed in the obstetrics list, how you word a problem greatly influences interpretation and defense. I remind you that if it is best to call a rose a rose, then do so.

If you choose to be generic however, you must have a sprinkling of the specifics, so the examiner can deduce what you mean by routine care. Using the above example of HMB - on some scattered patients, you might list specific treatment of progesterone, OCPs, IUD, DMPA, or GnRH agonists. For the most part, it's clear on what you mean by hormonal or medical therapy. IF he wants further details, he can ask you.

One strategy is, for all your patients with the same problem, word the work up and treatment generically and vague, such as "diagnostic tests or routine care", to force the examiner to inquire. This works great if indeed the examiner chooses the case. However, it is risky, for if the examiner does not get time to validate the specifics, he is forced to assume you don't know. Besides, remember the initial directive in the *Bulletin* was that you must list sufficient information such that the examiner can figure out how you work up and manage patients. The *Bulletin* advises against such terms as "usual" and "standard".

We'll talk later about how to handle a situation where you performed two separate operations on the same patient within the same year, such as both a D&C, and then later, a hysterectomy. For nonsurgical conditions, the admission diagnosis is listed in the preoperative diagnosis column also.

You want to make it clear in the Preoperative Diagnosis column why you took the patient to the operating room and that the procedure performed was appropriate. If you simply list "ovarian cyst" as the preoperative diagnosis, the examiner doesn't know if it was appropriate to have performed a laparoscopy. The size of ovarian cysts must be recorded in centimeters in the preoperative diagnosis. Although not mandatory, I strongly recommend you further qualify the cyst by type (simple or complex), side (left, right, or bilateral) and tumor markers, if appropriate.

Likewise, you want to list a stage or grade for prolapse cases. If you simply list uterine prolapse, how does the examiner know if the procedure performed was adequate or overkill? I'm sure you will agree that the preoperative diagnosis of procidentia warrants support of the apex. So "vaginal hysterectomy" isn't sufficient. On the other hand, "VH with uterosacral suspension, TVT" satiates the examiner's concerns that the apex was well supported, as well as prophylactic support of the urethra will avoid post op urinary incontinence.

The *Treatment* should include all surgical procedures. It should also include primary non-surgical treatment if the patient was admitted, but not operated on. For example, your *Preoperative or Admission Diagnosis* is PID and your *Treatment* is parenteral antibiotics. Non-primary treatment should be listed in the preoperative or admission diagnosis column. Let's say this patient did not respond to antibiotics and you had to take her to the OR. In this setting, your *Preoperative or Admission Diagnosis* may state "PID, tubo ovarian abscess refractory to antibiotics" and the *Treatment* may be "exploratory laparotomy, lysis of adhesions, drainage of tubo ovarian abscess".

The pathologic diagnosis should support the preoperative diagnosis. For example, if the preoperative diagnosis is HMB secondary to leiomyomata (AUB-L), the pathology should verify a leiomyomatous uterus. Furthermore include only the pertinent pathology, not the entire pathology report, and list the offending organ first. In this example, list first the uterus, the weight in grams and simply list leiomyomata, and cervix benign. Don't torture the poor examiner with the pathologist's verbatim report and clutter and drag out your list with irrelevant minutia. You will quickly learn that your column is tight and word count is a premium.

Hysterectomy specimens must include the uterine weight in grams. This is critical to show the examiner how the size of the uterus affects your clinical and surgical decision making. This helps you - especially if you were able to do a vaginal hysterectomy on a uterus larger than 250 grams. Furthermore, everyone has a hysterectomy for fibroids, but their size dictates the route of hysterectomy, as well as questions regarding preoperative and intraoperative tricks on reducing blood loss.

In cases without tissue for histologic diagnosis, the final clinical diagnosis should be listed. For example, let's say your preoperative diagnosis is "chronic pelvic pain refractory to conservative measures". Your treatment is "operative laparoscopy", but you didn't remove any tissue. Thus you would report your clinical diagnosis, such as "endometriotic implants, dense pelvic adhesions" in the *Surgical Pathology Diagnosis* column.

The *Complications* column is subject to interpretation. You must list obviously significant complications, like a ureteral or bowel injury, and include blood transfusions. However, some strategic thought must go into just how much detail you feel is appropriate. Again, I wouldn't clutter your case list with insignificant events that didn't change the patient's outcome or hospital stay. So the fever that spiked the evening of surgery, but was gone within 24 hours, is probably irrelevant. However, quite the contrary if it occurred on POD #2 and you had to launch a workup and start parenteral antibiotics.

Don't be afraid of the Complications column. If you operate enough, of course you are going to have some complications, just hopefully not on every patient. However, it looks suspicious and deceptive if a case list is *void* of *any* complications. Don't even think of selectively (oops!) withholding that nightmare complication, say a death. ABOG does audit, and if you committed fraud, not only do you sit out of your exam for three years, but you must report this disciplinary action for *the rest of your career*!

Like the obstetrics list, the "#" refers to the sequential ordering for all patients from all hospitals, so every patient will have a unique number. This is what the examiner refers to when he says, "Tell me about patient # __ ". The *hospital* # refers to the sequential ordering of hospitals being reported from. For example, if you admit patients to two hospitals, then they will be Hospital A and B, respectively. The *patient* # refers to the sequential ordering of patients reported from a given hospital. So let's say you operate on two patients at two different hospitals. The first is #1, and her *hospital* # is "A", so her *patient* # is "A-1". Whereas the second patient is #2, and her *hospital* # is "B", so her *patient* # is "B-1".

As in the obstetrics list, check at the top of each case list page whether the source of each case was from *Post Residency Cases, Senior Residency Cases*, or *Fellowship Cases*. The *Days in the Hospital* is the arithmetic difference between date of discharge and date of admission. So if you did a D&C as an outpatient, her number of days in the hospital is zero. If your vaginal hysterectomy patient went home on POD#1, then her number of days in the hospital is one.

Be attentive to details and use precise and up-to-date terminology. For example, use the Bethesda system (SIL) for Pap smear nomenclature. Likewise, the use of "complex" or "simple" alone for endometrial hyperplasia is insufficient and does not influence its management, but the presence or absence of atypia does. Even better would be to use endometrial intraepithelial neoplasia (EIN) nomenclature. The term "fibroid" is acceptable slang, but is not as precise or sophisticated as the term "leiomyomata".

As for all the sections, complete the columns with as much information as needed to easily follow your thought process for patient management. You can later trim strategically. To facilitate this process, start once again with a narrative summary of the clinical issues.

Clinical Summary

Joyce Collins is a 42-year-old 2G/2P who complained of progressive HMB for the past one year. Her menses are monthly and last up to 7 days, whereas previously they lasted only 4-5 days. The second and third days of her periods are so heavy that she is homebound and must change both a simultaneous super tampon and overnight pad every one hour while awake. She denies breakthrough bleeding. She has also recently started to experience night sweats. Pelvic exam reveals an 8–10-week size uterus, with several irregular masses consistent with leiomyomata. The ovaries are of normal size.

She was initially treated with oral contraceptive pills (OCP). Although her night sweats resolved, she had minimal improvement in her HMB after three cycles. She chose conservative surgery and underwent a hysteroscopically guided fractional D&C. She had obvious submucosal leiomyomata, and the secretory pathology was consistent with OCP suppression. The D&C also failed to improve her HMB. Thus, she elected definitive therapy.

She was counseled on the various routes for hysterectomy, as well as the pros and cons for a prophylactic oophorectomy and/or salpingectomy. She elected for, and underwent a vaginal hysterectomy and opportunistic salpingectomy.

Initial ABOG Form Entry

Joyce Collins presents an uncommon case list quandary in that she had two procedures performed within the same year of case list collections. You can only count a patient once, as each patient must have a unique patient number. You may, however, list both procedures. You can count each procedure in the total cases column of the summary sheet, but can only apply one to a specific category.

See Example 3 on page 79. JC is listed once as #52, and is the only patient with this designator on the gynecology case list. Both the D&C and the vaginal hysterectomy are listed, but each encounter is separated by a deliberate demarcating space between texts. In other words, each encounter should stand alone, such that the preoperative diagnosis supports each treatment.

On the Summary Sheet, you need to decide which category you want to put her in. You have four category options - D&C, abnormal uterine bleeding, uterine myomas or vaginal hysterectomy. However you can only apply one. It's always advantageous to have as many vaginal hysterectomies as possible, so let's apply her to this category. So now the vaginal hysterectomy category will have one each in the total cases and total applied columns.

List of Office Patients

The office practice case list has evolved over the past several years. When the pathology slide section was dropped from the exam in the mid 1990s, the number of categories in the office practice case list was lengthened.

The managed-care-driven trend and CREOG's mandate to push obstetrics/gynecology to primary care resulted in further additions to the office practice case list. Then, in 2001, the office list blossomed to 41 categories. Not surprisingly, the new players were in primary care, and the obstetrics-related categories were deleted. Personally performed ultrasounds were also added.

To accommodate the longer list of categories, the number of representative patients was expanded from 40 to 60, but in 2004 it was scaled back to 40 again. The maximum number of patients in each category was scaled from four to three and, then once again, to the current two.

Well, the pendulum swung back as OB/GYN practitioners rebelled about being forced into primary care. Most were quite content to remain specialists in women's health. Furthermore, residency training took a squeeze. Since the length of the residency remained unchanged at four years, something had to give to accommodate this additional mandate for primary care training. Unfortunately, the OB and GYN rotations were trimmed. Not surprisingly, this new batch of residents was spread thin and they were not as skilled in the specialty areas. Thus, either the residency had to be lengthened or the primary care requirements had to be loosened. For now, the specialty won; thus, all the primary care topics remain, but the heavy emphasis on detail to the level of an internist has been lifted. Finally, the exam focus shifted back to what a gynecologist needs to know to screen, diagnose and refer to the internists.

The pendulum swung again, but in a different direction in 2012 when obstetrical topics made their debut. This is curious, as you would think this would be addressed on the OB rather than the Office list. However, laborists are not involved in antenatal management, so their obstetrics list ignored the antenatal care. Like most pendulums though, it swung back in the traditional direction, and in 2014 the OB topics were deleted. This is good, because too many inappropriately, but innocently, used OB patients to fulfill categories such as diabetes and hypertension. Remember, the Office list is really intended to address issues in non-pregnant patients.

Currently you must list 40 patients. There are now 36 categories as listed below, but make sure to check the *Bulletin* for the most updated list. You may list no more than two from any one category. Although it's difficult to use more than twenty five categories, I challenge you to use all 36 categories. Remember, you will be accountable for all the categories, even those for which you didn't list a representative patient.

Office Practice Categories

1. Abnormal cytology, colposcopy, and CIN
2. Benign pelvic masses
3. Breast diseases (benign and malignant)
4. Diagnosis and management of hypercholesterolemia and dyslipidemias
5. Disorders of menstruation (amenorrhea, dysmenorrheal, AUB)
6. Domestic violence
7. Endocrine diseases (diabetes mellitus, thyroid or adrenal disease)
8. Endometriosis: diagnosis and office management
9. Evaluation and management of acute and chronic pelvic pain
10. Evaluation & office management of Urinary and Rectal Incontinence
11. Family planning (contraception)
12. Galactorrhea
13. Genetic counseling
14. Geriatrics
15. Hirsuitism
16. Immunizations
17. Infertility evaluation & management
18. Lifestyle counseling (smoking cessation, obesity, diet, exercise, substance abuse)
19. Major medical diseases (respiratory, gastrointestinal, cardiovascular, hypertension)
20. Minor medical diseases (headache, low back pain, irritable bowel)
21. Medical management of ectopic pregnancy
22. Office surgery (biopsy, hysteroscopy, sterilization, LEEP)
23. Office evaluation & management of pelvic floor defects
24. Pediatric & adolescent gynecology
25. Perimenopause and Menopausal Care
26. PCOS
27. Preventive care and health maintenance
28. Psychiatric illnesses (depression, anorexia, bulimia)

29. Sexual assault
30. Sexual dysfunction
31. Sexually transmitted infections
32. Ultrasonography
33. Urinary Tract Infections
34. Uterine myomata
35. Vaginal disease
36. Vulvar disease
37. Uncategorized

For those unchosen categories, simply list the category on your case list and record "None observed". Remember, you cannot include any patients who appear on the hospital lists. Also include the total number of office ultrasounds that you personally performed in obstetric and gynecologic patients, as well as in other areas (e.g., abdominal, thoracic, pediatric).

Column confusion is the most common construction error on the office case list. The Results column is intended for the results of the treatment, NOT the result of the diagnostic procedure. Think about it. Why would you have to jump two columns over and then back again? For example, if the problem is a High Grade SIL Pap smear, then your diagnostic procedure is colposcopic directed biopsies, whose results (eg ECC negative, ectocervix CIN III) are listed within that diagnostic procedure column. The treatment is then a LEEP and the pathology (CIS margins clear) is listed in the results column.

This concept is better understood if you write it out. Grab a blank office case list sheet and fill in each of the columns. The premise is that we read from left to right and top to bottom. Again, if you list your results for your procedure in the results column, the reader has to read through the next column, which is the treatment column, to get to the results column. He now realizes he needs to disregard and block out the treatment column, and go back and reread the procedure to match up the results. Are you confused? You can bet the examiner reading this case list is also. Let's compound the problem. Let's put the results for both the procedures and the treatment in the Results column. Do you now see the confusion in trying to figure out what results match with what? Hopefully Examples 4 and 5 on pages 80 and 81 will help you avoid this common mistake.

It's not a show stopper if you made this mistake, since so many others have as well. However, it stands out, in a good sense, when you've done it right, as it gives an impression of attention to detail and methodical and meticulous patient management.

In both the obstetrics and gynecology sections, we discussed how you word a problem greatly influences interpretation and defense. I used the calling a rose a rose analogy. I advised using general terms only when you had a large number of same-kind cases. Since you cannot list more than two patients per category, this does not apply to the office. I remind you once again that the beginning of the *Bulletin* states that the case list must have sufficient information to understand the care provided.

Specifically, be specific. Don't use generic terms such as diagnostic labs, routine health maintenance or age-appropriate counseling, because they tell the reader absolutely nothing. I know your strategy is that you're trying to bait the examiner into asking for specifics. However, this totally backfires if he doesn't ask. You just lost an opportunity for a pass on that topic.

Recall the example of HMB for the gynecology example. You could have the same problem on the office case list. However, you would not want to list the generic medical therapy as the stand alone treatment. You would want to be specific, such as progesterone, OCPs, IUD, DMPA, or GnRH agonists.

Don't misinterpret this to mean you cannot use generic concepts. On the contrary, sometimes this can cleverly dodge an unwanted line of questioning. For example, use a generic term for a drug if you want to avoid discussing its specific contents; for example, hormone replacement therapy rather than Prempro. On the other end of the spectrum, you can use generic terminology to bait questions you do want to discuss, such as antibiotics rather than Cipro.

Unlike the obstetric and gynecologic sections, at least you have a choice in the selection of patients. Use this choice to your strategic advantage. Strategize the organization of the office list before you enter the first patient to focus your collection of patients. Approach this strategy as you would an investment. How much *risk* are you willing to incur?

For the low-risk, conservative type, choose categories and patients that typify your mode of practice and are textbook examples. The advantage is that your comfort zone and knowledge base are at their highest and will be the least affected by anxiety under the exam environment. The disadvantage is that you leave the door wide open for the examiners to choose which "oddities" and "aberrations" to your theme they wish to explore.

Another conservative, but disguised as speculative, approach would be to chose categories that are difficult for you. Remember, your case list is a legal cheat sheet. Perhaps you find it tough to pull out primary amenorrhea from your case list hat. This would be a perfect case to list because you'll have the work up and management right in front of you. Even if the topic arises on a different patient, you can flip back to this case to guide your recall.

A speculative, high-risk taker can bait the examiners by listing rare categories (e.g., sexual dysfunction, pediatric gynecology, primary care topics) or extremes within common categories (e.g., intrauterine insemination for infertility or Müllerian tract abnormality for amenorrhea). The likelihood that such "oddities" will pique the examiners interest and therefore limit them to your agenda is high. You will be prepared and thus, perform well. The disadvantage is that you still need to know the basics: thus, the overall preparation is more involved. Since you are also on the fringe, the examiner may have greater expectations.

Ideally your portfolio should be diversified. In other words, your case list should have a sampling of both types of patients. Keep in mind your strategic options as you begin to collect patients. It will be obvious which strategy you should incorporate for most categories and patients.

Because choice is involved, collection of patients in this section is the most prone to procrastination. Keep a list of all of the categories on your desk and begin to collect representative patients. Since you are limited to two patients per category, stop collecting further patients after you have gathered four names. To avoid an avalanche at the end, begin screening categories for definite "keepers" or "rejects" by six months (November or December). Similarly, three quarters, if not all, of the categories should be chosen in the following three months (by February or March). If you have not already finished, only the remaining one quarter needs to be completed in the final three months.

For the four "keepers" in each category, write a narrative of the patient management issues. Next, extract the pertinent data for entry onto the ABOG form. Err on the side of entering too much information initially. It is easier to delete extraneous facts than to search later for incomplete or forgotten details.

Finally, you're supposed to list the number of office visits that were required to address each problem. This column is irrelevant, yet if you try to carry a problem from start to finish, it looks like you order a bunch of labs. A classic example is in diagnosing and managing PCOS. Although you truly may have ordered your labs in batches, if you list the problem from beginning to end, you'll have a long list of UPT, TSH, Prolactin, Testosterone, DHEA-S, 17-OHP, lipids, insulin and perhaps even more. The appearance is that you have absolutely no idea what to order, so you'll order everything in hopes that something is positive to point you in the right direction.

Instead address only one stage of the work up at a time. In the above PCOS saga, pick up the problem that she already has PCOS and her complaint is hirsuitism. Then the only appropriate labs would be Testosterone, DHEA-S and perhaps 17-OHP. You want to appear focused and deliberate with each step of your work up and treatment.

Clinical Summary—Conservative

Joyce Lauden is a 48-year-old 4G/4P who complains of night sweats, mood swings and irritability. She had a vaginal hysterectomy three years ago for heavy menstrual bleeding. Her physical exam and past medical history are unremarkable. She has no personal or family history of gynecologic malignancies. Your diagnosis is perimenopause. You advise her to try an estradiol patch 0.1mg twice weekly. Her symptoms resolve. For the initial ABOG form entry, see Example 6 on page 82.

Clinical Summary—Speculative

Jennifer Schroeder is a 21-year-old 1G/1P, who had an uncomplicated vaginal delivery 18 months ago. She complains of persistent unilateral galactorrhea. She discontinued the OCP 6 months ago, but still has not started her menses. She denies headaches or visual changes. A urine pregnancy test is negative. She has a progestin withdrawal bleed. Thyroid function tests are normal. The prolactin level is moderately elevated (65). A prolactin-secreting adenoma is diagnosed. You recommend an MRI or CT of the sella turcica to determine whether it is a micro- or a macro-adenoma. Because she is financially strapped, you settle for an x-ray, which is normal. She is started on bromocriptine, 1.25 mg q.h.s. x 1 wk, then increased to 2.5 mg b.i.d. A repeat prolactin test is normal, and her menses returns. For the initial ABOG form entry, see Example 7 on page 82.

Your office practice case list should have a variety of styles, ranging from conservative to speculative. The key is to tailor the style which is the most appropriate for each case.

Peer Review

By this point, you have become intimately entwined in the nitty-gritty details of each case. You know them almost too well. Not surprisingly, most of us cannot see the forest for the trees. For this reason, it is imperative to enlist the aid of others who can see the big picture. I recommend that you tap into a variety of resources, including specialists, generalists, academicians, non-academicians, peers who know you well, and peers who don't know you at all.

If you are a generalist, it is extremely helpful to seek a specialist's opinion and vice versa. The specialist will more likely reflect the profile of the examiner, and the generalist will be more familiar with the basic ACOG standards. Regardless, both sides quickly forget the other's unique perspective, especially if practicing in an exclusive environment. You want to critique your case list from as many angles as possible to best anticipate potential questions.

I recommend that you send your obstetrics section to a generalist and/or your referring maternal/fetal medicine specialist; the gynecology section to a generalist, your referring gynecologic oncologist and/or female pelvic medicine specialist; and the office practice list to a generalist and/or reproductive endocrinologist and/or family practitioner or internist. In addition, send one or more sections to someone who is familiar with your mode of practice (e.g., your partner or local colleague) as a check for consistency and conformity to your known mode of practice. Finally, send segments to a peer of like profile (e.g., another generalist or same specialty), who is less known to you to look for glaring mistakes and to evaluate adherence to the ACOG standard of care. A final check can be a professional, like faculty at a review course, who routinely reviews many case lists.

Remember to give your consultants ample time to review their sections. You must send the sections in sufficient time, but make your deadlines crystal-clear. Send the first batch in May or early June and have it due mid June or no later than July 1. Return revised drafts to them by the second week in July, with a due date in the third week of July.

The purpose at this time is to make recommendations for strategic organization of your case list. Return the masterpiece in August or September to help plan its defense. It is ideal, but not essential, to tap into all of the above resources. It is imperative to at least consult a few. Remember, their job is to give you guidance. You may want to incorporate all, some, or none of their recommendations. Take their advice for what it's worth, but make it worth your while!

Case List Logistics

Your case list must conform *exactly* to the ABOG specifications. You will download the instructions for preparing the case list after receipt of your application and fee. Keep it and the *Bulletin* readily at hand, for you will refer to them frequently. Do not rely on previous instructions, because instructions change yearly. Check and double-check for compliance each step of the way.

You absolutely—no ifs, ands, or buts—must duplicate the *exact* format of the ABOG forms. You can simply make copies of the original forms and then type in the data. The disadvantage is that this old-fashioned way makes editing difficult and almost always necessitates retyping the whole darn page to make it look acceptable. I recommend instead, that you use a computer with a program that *exactly* reproduces the ABOG form. You can either customize your own program (see Appendix D) or use the ABOG case list software.

The case list must be typed in 10-point font in a landscape view on 8.5 x 11 inch, unbound white paper. The headings must conform in all details, and you must provide the information indicated by the ABOG format.

Your name and case list number must be on every page. You need to identify if you are using senior residency, fellowship, or post residency cases. All case lists must be de-identified as required by the HIPAA privacy rule or they will be rejected. If you do not have patients to report in a category at each hospital, still insert the appropriate form in the proper order and specify "None" on the form. This also serves as a reminder that you are accountable for all the categories, not just the ones that you selected.

Each section must group overall headings in accordance with the following ABOG dictum:

1. Obstetrical Case List

   A. Number of Uncomplicated Spontaneous Deliveries—enumerated on page
   B. Obstetrical Categories—starts on page 1
   C. Total number of ultrasound and color Doppler examinations performed by you upon hospitalized obstetrical patients—enumerated on last page
   D. Total number of
      i. Apgar scores 5 or less
      ii. Infants <2500 grams
      iii. Perinatal deaths—Enumerated on last page

2. Gynecological Case List
   A. Gynecological Categories (1-30)—Starts on page 1
   B. Total number of ultrasound and color Doppler examinations performed by you upon hospitalized gynecological patients – enumerated on last page
3. Office Practice Case List
   A. Office Practice Categories—starts of page 1
   B. Total number of ultrasound and color Doppler examinations on
      i. Obstetrical patients
      ii. Gynecological patients
      iii. Other areas such as abdominal, thoracic, pediatric, etc.— Enumerated on last page

Standard nomenclature should be used. *Only* ABOG-approved abbreviations are acceptable (see Appendix A). Practically speaking, it's OK to use well-accepted abbreviations (i.e. HCG for Human Chorionic Gonadotropin). Your non-local reviewer should pick up on local abbreviations that are not universal and therefore should be deleted (e.g. IOL, Induction of Labor). Only the English language is permissible.

The pages of the case list should be numbered consecutively within each section, so each page has a unique number. Likewise, all patients must be numbered consecutively so each patient also has a unique number. For the Obstetrics and Gynecology lists, the hospital number refers to the sequential ordering of hospitals. The summary sheet must contain the combined totals of all hospitals. The affidavit sheet must be signed by the medical records librarian from *each* hospital. The case list must be arranged in the following order and submitted in triplicate (3 copies) and unbound:

A. Summary sheet (7 copies)
B. Affidavit sheet for each hospital
C. Obstetric patient list for each hospital
D. Gynecologic patient list for each hospital
E. Office patient list

Although your case list is not due until August 1, you will usually be notified in July as to the month of your exam. Theoretically, ABOG could later disapprove your case list, but this is uncommon. They will inform you of the exact date and time one month prior to your exam.

When you report for your exam, you must bring one *unaltered* copy of your case list. In 2008, candidates were allowed to bring a copy of the case list that had the patient's initials. Subsequently, this language has appeared only episodically in the letter notifying you of the date and time of your exam. Thus, make sure you double check to see if this is permissible. To be on the safe side, I suggest you bring a copy of both the de-identified list that you originally submitted, as well as one with patient's initials. You do not want to show up with the patient's initials list only, and discover that it is unacceptable that year, as you would be sent home. You must also sign a statement on the morning of the exam attesting that you have had no restrictions in your hospital privileges or medical license.

Strategic Organization of the Case List

The case list is the only exam component that you are allowed to complete ahead of time. As with any take-home test, you are empowered to polish it entirely to your standard. You have the luxury to strategize its organization and compose it to your advantage.

Strategy and tactics are defined as the purposeful and deliberate carrying out of intent. Most of us are familiar with these terms as they apply to the military. Strategy is the "why" or intent, and tactics are the "how to" or the steps to carry out the intent. Strategy and tactics are the root of the basic war dogma, "Know your enemy". To order troops to "take that hill" without regard to strategy and tactics would result in disaster. Battles are won on paper; they are simply fought on land, air, and sea. In other words, the battle is carefully studied from all angles to ensure victory before the first soldier bears arms.

Your best weapon on this test is your case list. Carefully inspect it from all angles to best plot your strategy. Then employ all necessary tactics to ensure victory. The first step in analyzing the "enemy" is to understand the reason for the case list. The purpose is to examine your ability to manage patients. You are held to the level of a consultant for non-Ob/Gyn physicians. Your strategy is to construct a case list that resoundingly reflects your understanding of this expectation.

As long as the case list meets the ABOG requirements, you have considerable freedom to incorporate your strategy. Numerous tactics can be used. The following is by no means all-inclusive, but rather should serve as a catalyst to help you develop your own strategy.

First, take a stance on the detail of your case list. ABOG states that "only pertinent data, not summaries", should be included. Nonetheless, a case list "insufficient in breadth and depth of clinical difficulty" may not be accepted. Furthermore, carelessly prepared or incomplete case lists may contribute to failure of the exam. On the other hand, exhaustive details leave little room for basic management questions and force the examiner to interrogate about trivia. Thus, the theme for completing the forms is analogous to the advice given to medical students for cutting sutures on their surgical rotations. "Not too long, not too short—just right!" Of course, each staff had a different preference; therefore, the poor student was always wrong! It wasn't long before the student figured out to ask the resident the staff's preference before each surgery.

Use the same strategy to tackle your case list. Obtain case lists from previous candidates. Note that there are as many different styles as there are candidates. Furthermore, the depth of information varies with each patient. There is, however, a bell-shaped curve representative of the depth of detail for each case list.

The following examples typify "too long" and "too short" and "just right" detail for <u>most</u> cases. I underscore most because clearly there are exceptions. Strategically, you want some cases at the extremes of the bell-shaped curve.

A "just right" case should project a logical sequence of sound patient management consistent with ACOG standards. The detail either satiates the examiner's need to ask questions or invites a discussion of routine, straightforward topics along any entry of the management algorithm. The theme is "bottom-line up front". Ideally, the majority of your case list is composed of such cases.

In Example 8 (page 82), note that the preoperative diagnosis of an "acute abdomen, but hemodynamically stable" justifies initial use of laparoscopy rather than laparotomy in this surgical emergency. Furthermore, the "suspected cornual pregnancy" was indeed confirmed; thus, the candidate prudently and humbly put down the laparoscope and proceeded with the laparotomy. His surgical decision to resect the cornual ectopic was consistent with the standard of care and the pathology further supported his preoperative suspicion.

The examiner's questions about the candidate's surgical management of ectopic pregnancy should be answered. If the examiner chooses to ask any questions, they would be generic and related to any step of the algorithm of ectopic pregnancy management. Furthermore, the examiner would probably confine his questions to the basics rather than explore esoteric spin-offs not addressed by the patient (e.g., medical management, risk factors, recurrence).

A "too long" case can block questions like a "just right" case, but differs in the degree of detail. A "too long" case has excessive detail, so the few remaining questions are at the end of the spectrum of patient management, dealing with the obscure and little known. A "too long" case list reflects an obsession with minutia that raises doubt of your ability to see the big picture. Suspicion also arises that the patient is subjected to extraneous and unnecessary lab tests and procedures.

The patient in Example 9 (page 83) is listed under the office category of *Perimenopausal and Menopausal Care;* yet other non-pertinent issues are raised and are therefore fair game for the examiner to address. Enumeration of implied tasks such as "history and physical exam", as well as the conventional screens of "Pap smear, mammogram and Hemoccult" suggests that the candidate may view them as mandatory for any menopausal patient. Not all of the diagnostic procedures are necessary in every case. No doubt this raises questions of the candidate's ability to recognize basic management issues. Finally, listing brand names of medications mandates justification of the specific brand and hence knowledge of its pharmacology. These unwelcomed questions can be avoided entirely by referring instead to the class of drugs (e.g., hormone replacement therapy instead of Premarin and Provera).

On the other hand, "too long" cases can be used to your strategic advantage if they occur sparingly throughout the case list (see Example 10 on page 84). They might block questions on a topic the candidate would rather not discuss. They can also be used as a legal crib sheet for a topic that is not easily remembered. The candidate can flip to the representative patient when the topic arises, even if not specifically discussing that patient.

As in the previous example, there are few unanswered questions. The remaining questions are on the fringe and beyond what would be expected for this topic. The candidate clearly followed a logical progression down the workup algorithm. Unlike the previous example, all of the ordered lab tests were necessary. Furthermore, referral to a specialist underscores the candidate's recognition that he or she has reached the extent of his or her abilities and humbly refers the patient's care.

In contrast to a "too long" case, a "too short" case provides insufficient information and obliges the examiner to inquire further. Because minimal information is provided, the examiner can start anywhere on the spectrum of questions. The scarcity of detail also leaves doubts about the thoroughness and compulsiveness of the candidate's management. If the bulk of the list exhibits such cases, the examiner is overwhelmed and frustrated as to where to start because there are questions on every case.

In Example 11 (page 85), the entire page leaves questions about every patient. The information is so sparse and generic that the examiner could spend the allotted time interrogating the candidate about this page alone. Imagine how the examiner will feel if this page is representative of the entire list! Pity the poor unsuspecting candidate who must face an examiner who is poised for attack.

If, however, "too short" types occur rarely on your case list, the candidate can bait the examiner to open discussion of a topic that the candidate wants to discuss. Because the information is sparse, the examiner most likely will start at the beginning and say, "Tell me about this patient." At this point, the candidate is in the driver's seat.

Like the previous example, Example 12 (page 86) leaves many questions unanswered. Note, however, that this topic is unusual, far from the mainstream "bread-and-butter" topics. It is strategically worded so that the only logical question is to start at the beginning: "What happened?" or "How did this patient present?" The candidate's control of the opening question drives subsequent ones that the candidate anticipated and is well prepared to answer. Note also that the candidate can buy a lot of time while scoring big.

On the same theme of volume is the concept of redundancy in the office practice case list. Remember, this is the only one of the three sections for which you can choose the patients. Recall also that you can list no more than two for each category.

I often will see candidates list essentially the same case, but two different patients for one category. For example, in the vaginal discharge category, you list two patients, each with yeast vaginitis—same problem, same procedure, same treatment, of course the same result as both got better. I am stumped with this strategy. Is it because you really want to talk about this topic? How exciting are two yeast infections? I think it is a waste of a patient and category, and also gives a cookie cutter impression.

If you're going to chose two patients for the same category, I recommend they be two different themes within that category. Go back to our vaginal discharge example - at least make one patient with acute candidiasis and the other chronic. Better yet, choose two completely different discharges—say one with yeast and the other with trichomonas or bacterial vaginosis.

In addition to the volume of data, there is considerable strategy in the wording of cases. Tailor each case to your objective. For example, on the obstetrics case list, you may elect to simply list "routine hemorrhage management" in the treatment column for the complication of postpartum bleeding. This wording is generic and therefore begs a general question; whereas if the treatment was more extreme (such as culminating in a hysterectomy), you may want to be specific to justify why you elected that modality of therapy. Remember, you never want to go generic if this is your only representative category.

Another similar debate is with the wording for fetal distress. I'm sure you know that "fetal distress" as an antepartum complication is outdated and a medico-legal no-no. Furthermore, the Category I, II, III fetal heart rate tracing nomenclature has replaced "non-reassuring fetal heart rate tracing" or "fetal intolerance to labor". Exceptions would include clarifying a modality of treatment. For example, use "terminal bradycardia" for an emergent operative delivery, or "fetal tachycardia" for chorioamnionitis. Likewise, your treatment for any of the above could generically be listed simply as "intrauterine fetal resuscitation". Although sometimes you may want to specify if you performed maternal position changes, fetal scalp electrode, fetal scalp stimulation or an amnio-infusion.

After you're satisfied with the volume, categories and wording for each case, consider the order in which to list the patients. ABOG mandates that you group like patients together under each separate category. The disadvantage is that the examiner can search out the worst or most complicated patient within each category in just seconds. The ABOG software will also list the patients in the chronological order that you entered them. Commercial software lists the categories alphabetically. Neither of these approaches takes advantage of strategic placement within each section.

The best placement of categories and the cases within a category is that which achieves your strategic goal. There will be a lot of moving and shaking in your case list and the construction will be in constant flux. It's not obvious as to which is the best placement until after you've entered all your cases.

A classic example is hysterectomy. If you listed your categories alphabetically, you would start page *one* of your GYN list with "Abdominal hysterectomy, any type (e.g. total, subtotal, laparoscopic, robotic")." "Vaginal hysterectomy" would be on the *last* page of your case list. This is disastrous, as both ACOG and ABOG clearly opine that vaginal hysterectomy is the ideal route. So the disgruntled examiner must muddle through all the other GYN categories before he finally makes it to vaginal hysterectomy.

The entire time, the examiner is saying "why not a VH?" for any non-vaginal routes. Unfortunately, his sour impression can't be easily undone when he finally stumbles on to VH on the last page. A simple cut/paste action can undo all your woes. *Start* your GYN list with "Vaginal hysterectomy". Voilà. Talk about a great first impression!

Put your best foot, or at least case, forward. In other words, list your best cases first under their respective category. What the heck! Why not strategically **bold**, CAPITALIZE, or *italicize* key words to catch the examiner's eye so he doesn't miss them?

Note carefully that a *best* case is not necessarily synonymous with flawless management and perfect outcome. *Best* implies a case that you know cold and are the best prepared to defend. A best case may be a case from hell, but it demonstrates your flexibility, quick thinking, humbleness in calling for help, or acknowledging error and henceforth changing a mode of practice.

A seasoned examiner will not be fooled by any order of listing of patients. Regardless of their location, know your worst cases best. Obviously, spread them out, with an ideal limit of one per page. Try not to put similar complications close together to avoid their jumping out on a skim-through. The exception is a recurrent complication that finally motivated you to change your mode of practice. Make it clear that you tracked the outcomes, recognized the redundancy of your error, and fixed it with resulting good outcomes.

All case lists should have some poor outcomes or complications. No one is perfect. As a matter of fact, a case list lacking an occasional complication is highly suspicious for willful withholding and may prompt ABOG to verify its authenticity.

Fraudulent case lists result in suspension from the exam. That's bad, but the worse part is that it will follow you the rest of your career. Remember, every single time you renew your medical licenses or hospital privileges you are asked, "Has there ever been any disciplinary action taken against you?" Remember also that you had your medical records director sign a notarized copy verifying the authenticity of your case list. This will also reflect poorly on your admitting hospital. Bottom line: don't even think about withholding any cases. You will woefully regret it your entire career.

In conclusion, the time spent to strategize the organization and construction of your case list is enormous. Certainly, it is logistically easier to list the patients chronologically or to let the computer program dictate their order. But the potential gain in strategizing is far greater than the time invested, as repeatedly confirmed by previous candidates reflecting on what they would do differently. A resounding response is "Construct my case list better". For they know, as will you know come August 1, that your case list is cast in stone.

Editing

Although the time frame for when the case list is due (August 1) relative to when its compilation is completed (June 30) is tight, there is time for at least one revision and perhaps more. One of the biggest regrets of previous candidates is running out of time to better organize and edit their case list. A strategically composed case list is by far easier to defend than a case list haphazardly thrown together. Besides, a mere six weeks of intense effort is minute compared with the year invested in its compilation.

Implementing your strategy during the compilation of the case list maximizes the efficiency of editing. However, the gestalt of the case list is not obvious until the first written draft. Critique the case list from the examiner's viewpoint. Look at it first from a distance, then up close. Your peers should afford you the same favor. The easiest facet of editing the big picture is the physical layout. Make sure it is reader-friendly. Esthetics that appease the reader's eye include the following:

1. Use a conventional, easy to read, font in sharp, dark, black ink.
2. The letters should be large enough to avoid eye strain (10-point font). Remember, many of your examiners wear bifocals. An average page has 4–6 patients (see Examples 13 and 14 on pages 87 and 88).
3. The layout should enable readers to delineate between cases and assist them in following the flow of management within each case. This is facilitated by:
   - Highlighting or shadowing category headings (see Example 15 on page 89)
   - Leaving space between separate thoughts within a case (See Example 16 on page 90)
   - Placing vertical tracking lines to demarcate columns
   - Placing horizontal tracking lines to follow flow within and between columns (See Example 17 on page 91)

- Placing bullets to align flow of thought (See Example 18 on page 92)
  - The most common bullet is a circle o, although it can be a hyphen- , asterisk*, squiggle~, etc.
  - Bullet on the right should match the bullet on the left
  - If there is only one word for the problem or treatment, then it does not need a bullet
- Capitalization: ALL to emphasize or for abbreviations (eg. LIGATION of the URETER or TAH) (See Example 19 on page 93)
  - Capitalize the first letter in the lead word of a grouping (Chronic pelvic pain secondary to endometriosis (See Example 19 on page 93)
- No periods (this is not a sentence)
- Highlight, <u>Underline</u>, **Bold,** Shadow, Indent(See Examples 20, 21, 22 on pages 94, 95, and 96)

4. Verify that the mandatory objective data are included:
   - Within each section, the columns should contain the required information:
     - Summary Sheet: verifying that the numbers are correct.
     - De-identified hospital and patient #.
     - Check and list the appropriate heading: Post Residency Cases, Senior Residency Cases, or Fellowship Cases
   - Obstetrics
     - Unique case list # and page #
     - Gravida and parity only
     - EGA in whole numbers
     - Friedman terminology for dysfunctional labor, not FTP (optional) (see Example 23 on page 97)
   - Gynecology
     - Size (cm) of ovarian cysts
     - Surgical pathology weight of uterus (gm)
     - Bethesda terminology for Pap smear cytology and histology for biopsies (optional)

- Endometrial hyperplasia with or without atypia or Endometrial Intraepithelial Neoplasia (EIN) (optional)
- Leiomyomata, not fibroids (optional)
- Abnormal uterine bleeding or specifics (eg. PALM-COEIN system), not dysfunctional uterine bleeding (optional)
- Office practice
  - 40 patients total
  - Maximum of 2 patients per category
  - Do not duplicate patients that also appear on the Ob or Gyn lists.
- Laboratory values with appropriate units
  - Use ABOG-approved abbreviations only (see Appendix A)
  - No typographical errors
  - Minimize grammatical errors

Now step back and look for trends. To do so, answer the following questions:

1. Is your best foot forward? In other words, are your best cases listed first in each category?
2. Have you limited significant complications and worst cases to one per page?
3. Have you spread out like complications and avoided listing them consecutively?
4. Does each page have a variety of patient management themes?
5. Does each page vary in complexity?
6. Is the case list mode of practice consistent with how you actually practice?

Finally, get out the microscope and analyze each case for the following:

1. Can the examiner clearly follow your flow of patient management? (see Examples 24 and 25 on pages 98 and 99). This is especially paramount on the obstetrics and office list where column confusion makes all the difference. Refer again to Example 1 on page 78 and Examples 4 & 5 on pages 80 and 81. Additionally, each topic on the obstetrics case list should be organized chronologically, and the management of each topic should flow from left to right. In other words, the reader should see problem "A" in the antepartum column and see the matching treatment directly to the right in the operative

procedures and/or treatment column. If problem "A" occurred first in the pregnancy, then it should be listed before problems that developed later.
2. Are the majority of cases "just right" in volume (pertinent data, not summaries)? (see Example 26 on page 100)
3. Are there only a few "too long" and "too short" cases? Do they meet your strategic objective?
4. Do all cases meet the ACOG standard of care? If not, justify why.
5. How does the wording generate topics? Is it consistent with your intended strategy?

If you have followed each of the above steps, your case list is ready to submit.

Although theoretically, each draft can be edited, the impact declines exponentially with the number of editions beyond two. Furthermore, the clock is ticking and time will be up. Push for at least one rewrite. Two edits are ideal, but difficult, given the time constraints. Nonetheless, a comparison of your original draft with your masterpiece makes all of the time and effort well worth the blood, sweat, and tears. After all, better now than after the test.

Using the Case List as a Study Tool

You must know your case list *cold* to pass the exam. This dogma is steadfastly affirmed by successful candidates. One way to meet this mandate, as well as tackle your list of study topics (see Chapter 8), is to organize your studies around your case list. There will be some overlap of topics; therefore, this system is not as time-intensive as it initially seems.

First, obtain three large three-ring binders—one for each of the three sections. Then for every patient, draft a narrative summary of the management issues as if you were presenting her at morning report or teaching rounds. Examples for each of the three sections of the case list were cited earlier (see pages 41-53). Next, for each OB patient, file her prenatal record and delivery notes; for each GYN patient, file her H&P and operative report; and for all hospitalized patients, file the discharge summary.

Now identify the issues that are raised by this case, and couple each topic with the pertinent reference(s) from the *ACOG Compendium* and the *Pearls of Exxcellence*. Try to limit your review to these resources. It is a rarity that the Compendium does not have a reference on a topic. In this case, check next the *ACOG Precis* and as a last resort, other references. Be disciplined and extract only relevant issues. File these behind the hospital records.

Finally, put yourself in the examiner's shoes and brainstorm what questions may be asked. Consider questions directly related to each patient as well as spin-off topics. Verify your hunches by cross-referencing topics raised by your peers and especially in mock oral exams.

Here is an example of how to use your case list as a study tool:

Case list—Patient No. 124 (Example 26 on page 100)

Clinical summary: L.V. is a 30-year-old 2G/1P whose pregnancy was complicated by maternal obesity and a 40-lb weight gain. An ultrasound obtained at 38 weeks estimated fetal weight of 4000 grams. Her first stage of labor was 8 hours, and her second stage was 45 minutes.

Primary clinical issue: Shoulder dystocia

Spin-off topics: Macrosomia, maternal obesity, weight gain in pregnancy, gestational diabetes, ultrasonography, dysfunctional labor, induction/augmentation of labor, FHR monitoring, Ob anesthesia, operative vaginal deliveries, and episiotomy.

ACOG Compendium references:
Shoulder Dystocia - Practice Bulletin; Operative Vaginal Delivery - Practice Bulletin; Fetal Macrosomia - Practice Bulletin; Induction of Labor – Practice Bulletin; Gestational Diabetes - Practice Bulletin; Obstetric Analgesia and Anesthesia - Practice Bulletin; Dystocia and the Augmentation of Labor - Practice Bulletin; Ultrasonography in Pregnancy - Practice Bulletin; Intrapartum Fetal Heart Rate Monitoring - Practice Bulletin, Pearls of Exxcellence; Fetal Heart Rate Abnormalities, Episiotomy - Practice Bulletin.

You have accomplished many goals by this tactic. No doubt you now know the patient cold! You have also reviewed at least ten topics that surely were on your study list. Finally, your brainstorming of potential questions has better enabled you to defend your management or to discuss related topics.

Defending Your Case List

Forewarned is forearmed. In other words, preparedness is your best defense. For this exam, ideal preparedness implies that the examiner actually asks the questions that you predicted. The challenge is to determine which questions the examiner will ask. Remember, the purpose of the case list is to examine your ability to manage patients. This requires validating your knowledge of the basic clinical sciences, but especially your ability to apply that knowledge to the practice of medicine. You know your case list better than anyone. Hence, you are probably the toughest critic of all. **If you were the examiner, what questions would you ask?**

To prepare your defense, step into the examiner's shoes. Pick up someone else's case list and look at it. Note that after just a few minutes you already have an image of its owner. The components of the first impression based on your case list are no different from the components in meeting someone.

Surprisingly, the bulk of the first impression is based on appearance. In other words, "it's not what you say, but how you say it". The case list's first impression is based on its physical layout and organization. Of course you can't judge a book by its cover. Therefore, the examiners will then peruse the list for generalities to get a feel for the candidate's mode of practice and whether it conforms to the ACOG standard of care. Finally, the examiners will select individual cases for questioning to validate their hunches.

Now tackle your case list with these three components in mind: first impression, general themes/trends, and specific cases that stand out. A formula for this process is described in the previous discussion of editing. Obviously the best defense is to organize the list strategically, so it best withstands the brunt of the examiners' offense. Once the case list is submitted however, it is set in stone. Now you must defend "the writing on the wall". This is how.

Start by determining your case list's first impression. The Summary Sheet is the most telling for the obstetrics and gynecology sections for a number of reasons. The volume of patients within each category is the most revealing element. The numbers indicate experience, complication rate, mode of practice and adherence to the ACOG standard of care.

In the obstetrics section, the total number of deliveries, which is the summation of total cases and total uncomplicated spontaneous deliveries, reveals how busy you are. The average number of deliveries is 75–150. Significant deviation, such as <50 or > 200, raises concern that you are either not busy enough or too busy to optimally maintain your technical skills and clinical judgment. You must have a ready explanation to justify the extremes (e.g., > 200—MFM specialist, joined a busy practice; < 50—started a rural solo practice, extended maternity leave).

Next, calculate your primary and repeat cesarean section rate. The summary sheet no longer has a category just for this, so it takes a motivated examiner to extrapolate the numbers. Make it easy and be ready for him.

Chapter 5 • The Case List

You also must be able to defend your math (the components of the denominator). Although the national cesarean section rate is about 30-35%, the average rate on most case lists is 20-35%. Significant deviation such as < 10% or > 50% may prompt inquiry into your judgment in criteria selection for cesarean delivery. Justify exceptional rates (e.g., > 30%-MFM at a tertiary center with preterm deliveries or no VBACs in a rural setting secondary to lack of anesthesia availability or maternal requests for elective CDs; <10%-low-risk obstetrics practice in a rural setting).

The remaining rates that can be calculated have less defined values. Examples include VBAC and induction rates. As noted above, extremes are a red flag. Traditionally too few VBACs were a red flag. Given the increasing complications of vaginal deliveries after a prior cesarean delivery, the pendulum is swinging back in favor of elective repeat cesarean deliveries. A low VBAC rate may be a marker that the patient is counseled with prejudice to dissuade her from trying labor. Maybe you can't even offer VBACs due to the lack of availability of anesthesia. At the other end of the spectrum, a high elective induction rate is suspicious that convenience rather than sound medical indications, drive your decision making. Similarly, the number of vacuum or forceps deliveries is not eye-catching unless it is excessive. A random check verifies that they are used appropriately (e.g., rare mid-pelvic deliveries or rotations).

Few or no breech deliveries cue questions about the steps for a breech delivery. On the other hand, the national trend is to deliver breeches by cesarean section, in spite of ACOG's recent endorsement for vaginal breech deliveries. Thus, fewer than two vaginal breech deliveries trigger the examiner to scrutinize your competency to practice this fading art. Obviously, the safest route for both the mom and baby is a vertex vaginal delivery. Thus, expect questions on external cephalic versions: counseling, candidates, contraindications, techniques and success rates. A nice way to block this question is simply to make an annotation such as "failed/refused-declined/successful ECV" in the antepartum complications column.

A high number of obstetric ultrasounds may prompt questions about your technical proficiency and quality control measures. A quick glance at the Apgars below 5, perinatal deaths, and postpartum admission columns prompts a quick search in the case list for the corresponding case.

Attention to detail and precise terminology blocks out questions, scores points for style and satisfies the examiner's concern for a level of understanding on a topic. Under the abnormal fetal growth category, preface IUGR with symmetric or asymmetric. Simply listing a patient as a diabetic makes it impossible to determine if the care was appropriate; whereas specifying her White's classification eliminates ambiguity.

It's best to call a spade a spade. In other words, if your induction was truly elective, then word it accordingly in the antepartum complications column. Refer to Induction of Labor – ACOG Practice Bulletin for ACOG appropriate indications for induction. Impending/suspected macrosomia as an indication for induction, although commonplace, lacks evidence and will only get you into a miserable discussion of scientific interpretation of the literature as well as trying to justify a breach of ACOG standard of care.

You know the expected questions for certain topics, so just cut to the chase. In multifetal pregnancy, make sure to specify twins or other, the chorion and amnion status, and presentation at deliver (eg. vertex/vertex). On operative vaginal deliveries, absolutely specify outlet or low.

In perusing the gynecology section, the examiner will again first check the numbers. Reportedly, you must do at least ten of a particular procedure annually to maintain your skills. Historically, vaginal hysterectomies fall into this category for many candidates. This prompts the question, "Dictate the steps of a VH".

Similarly, the examiner will search the indications for your abdominal hysterectomies to make sure that they could not have been attempted vaginally in the first place. Some common reasons to support why the patient was not a VH candidate include: nulliparity, inadequate uterine decensus, contracted pelvis, prior multiple cesarean sections, enlarged uterus, history of PID or suspected endometriosis. Thus, make your wording clear in the preoperative diagnosis column to defend your indication for your route of hysterectomy. But check the parity and weights first to make sure you don't look silly. Specifically, to use the excuse of lack of decensus in a multiparous patient or to state the uterus was enlarged for uteri less than 200 grams will backfire on you.

On the same theme, you must be able to defend the indications for your laparoscopic assisted hysterectomies. First use the appropriate definitions for laparoscopic assisted vaginal hysterectomy (LAVH), laparoscopic supracervical hysterectomy (LSH) total laparoscopic hysterectomy (LSH) and robotic assisted hysterectomy. Hopefully your case list doesn't have all laparoscopic hysterectomies or you will look like a one-surgery-for-all surgeon. In 2016, ABOG astutely closed the loophole of tucking LAVHs, LSHs, and robotic assisted hysterectomies deceptively into the VH category by specifying these are to be included in the abdominal hysterectomy category.

The alarming complication rate and the national decline in residency training of vaginal surgery have sparked a national debate. The concern is that the LAVH is inappropriately substituted to compensate for inadequate vaginal surgical skills. The above list that excludes a patient as a VH candidate applies only partially to the LAVH patient. Lack of decensus or an inadequate pelvic outlet cannot be overcome by the laparoscope, unless you perform a LSH or TLH. A uterine specimen weight less than 200 grams does not support your contention that an enlarged uterus prohibited attempting a VH. It also raises doubt of your pelvic exam abilities. Furthermore, desire for a BSO should not be the only indication for an LAVH. A competent vaginal surgeon should be able to remove the ovaries at least 60-70% of the time. Only if you are unsuccessful should you complete the procedure laparoscopically. To subject the majority of patients to what applies only to the minority makes no sense and suggests that the surgeon lacks confidence.

Perhaps the best defense for a case list with a paucity of VH is honesty. Many of you were heavily trained in laparoscopy and robotic surgery. I would confess that in *your* hands, you are more comfortable and *safer* with the laparoscope or robot. That does not however, overshadow your understanding that a vaginal hysterectomy is the preferred route. Offer that you are seeking mentoring and hoping to enhance your skills. Additionally, suggest that you would freely refer the patient to a colleague proficient in VH.

Unless you have a predominance of vaginal hysterectomies, you can expect a question on your thought process for choosing the route of hysterectomy and how you counsel the patient on the risks/benefits/alternatives for each route. You're golden if your case list has a blend of all the types of hysterectomies.

The Council on Resident Education in Obstetrics and Gynecology (CREOG) mandated the inclusion of urogynecology in the Ob/Gyn residency training in the mid 1990s. Subsequently, ABOG has expanded the categories where urogyn questions can pop up: defects in pelvic floor, rectovaginal or urinary tract fistula, urinary and fecal incontinence (operative management) and urinary incontinence (medical management). Just the fact that these categories exist is justification alone to prompt a line of questions. So don't think you're off the hook if you don't have any patients in these categories.

A reasonable line of questioning is, "How do you support your vaginal cuff in a routine vaginal hysterectomy to prevent prolapse in the first place?" Of course, you can satiate the examiner's concern by simply listing this in your treatment column. So rather than listing only a vaginal hysterectomy, you may also include modified Mayo/McCall cul de plasty or uterosacral ligament shortening/suspension.

But the question doesn't end there. How does your approach change if the indication is procidentia? Be prepared for the examiner to give you his pen and ask you to draw your initial incision at the cervico-vaginal junction. The answer is anteriorly at the supra-vaginal septum at the cervico-vaginal junction since the ureters are saggy posteriorly in the setting of prolapse and at greater risk for injury.

Of course then, how are you going to support the apex in the setting of prolapse? Make sure you refer to ACOG Practice Bulletin <u>Pelvic Organ Prolapse</u>. The technique you use for a routine, non-prolapsed hysterectomy is not sufficient. Your options are uterosacral shortening and suspension, sacrospinous ligament fixation, abdominal colposacropexy, or a total vaginal mesh/graft. Brace yourself, as this may prompt questions on the surgical technique for the above options.

Along the lines of prolapse, you must be prepared for questions on incontinence, both urinary and fecal. You first need to describe the preoperative work up. The ACOG Practice Bulletin <u>Urinary Incontinence</u> does not support fancy multichannel urodynamic testing in the uncomplicated patient, so be prepared to discuss how a generalist can perform right there in the office.

The exam focus is how to treat and prevent urinary incontinence. You must be able to counsel the patient on her options. Absolutely you have to be able to describe in detail at least one of those procedures, including intraoperative and postoperative complications. If you truly don't perform these surgeries, call your local generalist or urogynecologist and observe these procedures. If you can see it in your minds eye, it will be so much easier to defend and especially to think on your feet during the exam.

Now you may really be wiggling in your seat about all these urogynecologic questions. You're a bit anxious, because you don't perform *any* of these procedures, since you appropriately refer them all to FPMRS. Don't worry, as you are not alone. The majority of case lists that I review don't have any urogynecology cases. However, since you are on the front lines, you must know how to screen, work up and make a diagnosis before you refer.

Another red flag is too many induced abortions. This finding is particularly worrisome for pregnancies greater than 12 weeks, especially if they are elective. As you can imagine, this is a delicate political topic. They will not question the ethics, rather they'll have questions about your technique.

Many of you generalists are appropriately no longer performing any oncology cases, since patient mortality is lower in the specialist's hands. Thus, I am seeing more case list with a big fat zero in the invasive carcinoma category for those practitioners in community hospitals who do not have an oncologist on hand. As a matter of fact, there are rare questions on staging.

So, as you may have guessed, this does not get you off the hook if you have no patients in this category. The shift now is making sure you don't get caught with your pants down. In other words, how do you carefully work up a patient to make sure you don't get to the OR and have the pathology come back with an unexpected malignancy? You must know the bread and butter cancers though - specifically cervical, ovarian and uterine.

In addition to the total number of procedures, other categories on the Summary Sheet are revealing. Examiners will search out hospital stays longer than 7 days. All they have to do is thumb down the Days in Hospital column. They can find the longer stays in a heartbeat, regardless of where they are hidden. Be prepared to defend why your patient required a lengthy hospital stay.

Other categories to be prepared for, even if you don't have any, are those with complications: post op fever, thromboembolism, urinary tract, GI, pain, neurologic and wound healing. You need to be able to recognize, work up and manage these complications. In 2008, preoperative evaluation of coexisting conditions (respiratory, cardiac, and metabolic diseases) made its debut. This again reflects that swing of the pendulum back to what does a gynecologist need to know about medical issues to not get caught with his pants down.

Note that all three sections require you to list the number of office and inpatient ultrasounds that you personally performed. This new statistic appeared in 2000. Feedback suggests that a high number is a red flag. If you perform obstetric ultrasounds, make sure you refer to ACOG Practice Bulletin <u>Ultrasonography in Pregnancy</u> and Committee Opinion <u>Performance and Interpretation of Imaging Studies by the Obstetrician/ Gynecologist.</u>

You should also be aware of the levels of obstetric ultrasounds and their components. Contrary to popular usage, there is no official terminology of a level I, II, or III ultrasound. Rather, the three levels are basic, comprehensive and limited. The components of a basic ultrasound include the following:

- Fetal number
- Fetal presentation
- Documentation of fetal lie

- Placental location
- Assessment of amniotic fluid volume
- Assessment of gestational age
- Survey of fetal anatomy for *gross* malformations
- Evaluation for maternal pelvic masses

A detailed or targeted ultrasound is performed and interpreted by specially trained personnel proficient in the detection and recognition of a physiologically or anatomically defective fetus. If you profess to be such an expert, expect technical questions about the specific components within the anatomic survey. On the other hand, know when it is judicious to offer a limited ultrasound only. Common reasons include the following:

- Assessment of amniotic fluid volume
- Fetal biophysical profile testing
- Ultrasonography-guided amniocentesis
- External cephalic version
- Confirmation of fetal life or death
- Localization of the placenta in antepartum hemorrhage
- Confirmation of fetal presentation

Similarly, if you perform gynecologic ultrasounds, be familiar with ACOG Technical Bulletin, <u>Gynecologic Ultrasonography</u>. The most common test topic is determining when to do a transvaginal vs. a transabdominal ultrasound. Secondly, be prepared to expound on which ultrasound features of an adnexal mass are characteristic of benign vs. malignant lesions. Bear in mind that ACOG does not support routine ultrasound screening for ovarian cancer. Finally, expect some technical questions about how to diagnose an ectopic pregnancy.

You must be prepared for questions about ultrasound technique and interpretation if you include ultrasounds in your summary sheet. It is highly likely that you will get some of the above questions if you performed both obstetric and gynecologic ultrasounds. Definitely be prepared to also discuss your quality control measures. On the other hand, if you don't have any ultrasounds reported, you can expect basic or generic questions, if any.

The Summary Sheet gives examiners the most bang for their buck because the facts are right in the open. Next they will hone in closer. They will skim through the case list to get a gestalt of the clinical style.

The physical layout and organization of the case list make the initial impression of your attention to detail. Examiners will conduct a quick check to see whether it is reader-friendly, organized and free of spelling and grammatical errors and whether it conforms to the ABOG requirements. The examiner's checklist is similar to the one described in the discussion of editing. Remember, the examiner receives your case list before he meets you, so don't underestimate the impact this makes and how it influences the examiner's questions.

The gynecologic section is the easiest to assay attention to detail. Examiners will search out your youngest hysterectomy. You will need to justify her hysterectomy, especially if her gravida and parity are low. The postoperative pathology should agree with your preoperative diagnosis. For example, if you performed a hysterectomy for abnormal uterine bleeding secondary to uterine leiomyomata and the postoperative pathology showed a normal uterus, you need to explain why. Likewise, hysterectomies for the mere presence of leiomyomata are not indicated. Justify the hysterectomy with complications from leiomyomata such as HMB unresponsive to hormonal therapy or D&C.

If you perform incidental appendectomies, you need to justify why. Expect questions about the anatomy and blood supply of the appendix and postoperative complications. On the same theme, an incidental hysterectomy during concurrent prolapse surgery is controversial. You can avoid this topic if you have an appropriate indication for the hysterectomy or if the patient at least also has symptomatic uterine prolapse. Finally, if you performed a procedure for chronic pelvic pain or an adnexal mass, be prepared to list the differential diagnosis.

After examiners have a feel for the case list, they will beeline for individual cases. The obvious red flag is a case with complications. Each examiner has his own agenda and style. Remember to think first of horses rather than zebras when you hear hoof beats. In other words, the examiner will most likely start at the top rather than the bottom of the patient management algorithm. Plan your defense accordingly. Approach each case as described earlier in the discussion of using your case list as a study tool (page 66). Identify the main patient management issue or "bottom-line up front". Prepare first for the obvious, then work your way down the flow chart. Save preparation for the esoteric for last, if at all.

Finally, I want to end where we started. I want to drive home the fact that your best defense is predicting your exam questions. Remember, defending your case list is only a half hour for each section. Although 30 minutes will seem like an eternity, it does limit the number of cases that can be covered regardless of the size of your case list.

Recall that the Structured Cases section is also 30 minutes. If there are five cases, this means each case is covered in about six minutes. Each case usually has at least three follow up questions, so about two to three minutes per question. The case list questions are not predetermined and follow up questions are often dictated by your answer to the previous question. Thus, it takes longer for the examiner to phrase his question. Back to the point that you have only 30 minutes - the examiner can only get through about ten (averaging three minutes/case) to fifteen cases (averaging 2 minutes/case). Knowing this, a skilled examiner will strategically review your case list to bring to the surface the top cases that carry the highest yield for him to judge if you're a pass or fail.

So with that in mind, I recommend you pick out the ten cases that you would ask about if you were the examiner. Better yet, ask at least three other colleagues the same question. We all have our own reasons for selecting those ten. Those reasons include: identifying cases with complications, a topic of personal interest, a challenging diagnostic dilemma, a technically difficult case, an unusual or esoteric subject - to name a few. Regardless the rationale, you will see that at least five of the same cases overlap on everyone's list. Most likely these are going to be on your examiner's list too.

So obviously, the more opinions and lists you gather, the better you will be able to fine tune those top ten cases. Once you narrow those down, dissect them from every angle. Again enlist your colleagues' help and come up with as many questions as possible. Surely you will then have thought of most of the same questions as the examiner.

Remember to confine your preparation to a review. The ACOG *Compendium* is the best resource to keep you on track. You are expected to demonstrate a level of knowledge similar to other board-certified obstetricians and gynecologists. Once you have reached this level, the examiner will move quickly to the next question.

No doubt, examiners will sometimes drive you beyond the pass threshold. They may want to explore your depth of understanding of a particular topic. More likely, they simply want to verify that you will acknowledge your limitations.

Lastly is a tool to review your case list systematically. Highlight common ground topics for all cases with a different color. Common ground topics would include the pathophysiology, etiology, or definition for a disease, work up (labs and radiology) and medications. For example, let's say you use green to highlight any medication on your list. This is your cue to then know the active ingredient or content for brand name or generic drug, mechanism of action, indications/ contraindications, dosing, side effects and antidote.

In conclusion, your best defense is to be prepared. Your first line of defense is a strategically constructed case list. Your main defense, then, is to be prepared for the questions you have anticipated. The secret is your accuracy in predicting these questions. The more your case list is critiqued and the more mock oral exams you take, the better your chances of uncovering likely questions. Thus, when it is finally exam time, you will be answering questions that you have already heard many times before.

Example 1 Confusion Complications Column

#	Pt # No.	Age	Gravida	Para	Gest. Age	Complications Antepartum	Complications Delivery or Postpartum	Operative Procedures and/ or Treatment	Days in Hosp.	Newborn Complications	Newborn Wgt.	Newborn Apgar 1 & 5 Minutes	Newborn Days in Hosp.
16	A16 284486024	27	4	3	38	AI GDM	Protracted labor Category II FHR	Routine diabetic care. Pitocin augmentation CD	3	None	3760	9/9	5

Example 2 Clinical Summary Extract and First Draft of ABOG Form

#	Pt & Hospital No.	Age	Gravida	Para	Gest. Age	Complications Antepartum	Complications Delivery or Postpartum	Operative Procedures and/ or Treatment	Days in Hosp.	Newborn Complications	Newborn Wgt.	Newborn Apgar 1 & 5 Minutes	Newborn Days in Hosp.
42	Karen Burke 652688	34	2	0	38	Chronic hypertension Superimposed severe preeclampsia Arrest of dilation	None	Anti-hypertensives Magnesium sulfate Misoprotol cervical ripening Pitocin induction Intrauterine press catheter Primary CD	4	None	3435	9 & 10	3

Example 3 Clinical Summary Extract and Initial Entry

#	Initials & Hosp. No.	Age	Gravida	Para	Diagnostics Preoperative or Admission (Include size of ovarian cysts	Treatment	Surgical Pathology Diagnosis (uterine weight in grams	Complications (Include blood transfusions)	Days in Hosp.
52	Joyce Collins	42	2	3	HMB unresponsive to hormonal therapy	Hysteroscopic-guided fractional dilatation and curettage	Endometrium-secretory Endocervix-benign	None	0
					Leiomyomata with HMB unresponsive to hormones and dilatation and curettage	Vaginal hysterectomy, bilateral salpingectomy	Uterus-200 grams Leiomyomata Cervix-benign Bilateral tubes-benign	None	1

Example 4   Office Column Confusion **WRONG WAY**

List of Office Practice Patients

Candidate's Name: *Post Residency Cases
Caselist Number: July 1, 200_ – June 30, 200_
                                                                                 Page 1

#	Age	Grav	Para	Problem	Diagnostic Procedures	Treatment	Results	Number of visits
1	28	2	2	HGSIL Pap smear	Colposcopy	LEEP	ECC – negative Ectocervix – CIN III CIS – margins clear	

Pass Your Oral OB/GYN Board Exam!

Example 5 Office Column Confusion **RIGHT WAY**

List of Office Practice Patients

Candidate's Name: *Post Residency Cases
Caselist Number: July 1, 200_ – June 30, 200_
                                                                                Page 1

#	Age	Grav	Para	Problem	Diagnostic Procedures	Treatment	Results	Number of visits
1	28	2	2	HG SIL Pap smear	Colposcopy ECC – negative Ectocervix – CIN III	LEEP	CIS – margins clear	2

Example 6 Clinical Summary—Conservative

#	Initials & Hosp. No.	Age	Gravida	Para	Problem	Diagnostic Procedures	Treatment	Results	No. of Visits
	Joyce Lauden	48	4	4	Vasomotor symptoms Mood lability	None	Hormone replacement therapy	Resolution of symptoms	3

Example 7 Office Practice Clinical Summary Speculative

#	Initials	Age	Gravida	Para	Problem	Diagnostic Procedures	Treatment	Results	No. of Visits
	J.S.	21	1	1	Secondary amenorrhea, galactorrhea	Urinary pregnancy test (normal) Progesterone challenge (withdrawal bleed) Thyroid-stimulating hormone (normal) Prolactin level (elevated) Coned x-ray sella turcica (normal)	Oral contraceptive pills Bromocriptine	Prolactin-secreting pituitary micro-adenoma Return of menses Repeat prolactin (normal)	3

Example 8 "Just Right"

#	Initials & Hosp. No.	Age	Gravida	Para	Diagnosis Preoperative or Admission	Treatment	Surgical Pathology Diagnosis	Complications	Days in Hospital
	CM 496264	27	5	2	Acute abdomen, hemodynamically stable Ectopic pregnancy, (suspected cornual)	Laparoscopy Laparotomy Wedge resection of left cornua	Cornual ectopic pregnancy	None	1

Example 9   "Too Long" — The Wrong Way

#	Initials	Age	Gravida	Para	Problem	Diagnostic Procedures	Treatment	Results	No. of Visits
	J.L.	48	4	4	Night sweats Mood lability Hypermenorrhea Smoker Obese Decreased libido	History and physical exam Pap smear Mammogram Hemoccult screening Bone densitometry Endometrial biopsy (Dyssynchronous endometrium) Estradiol FSH, LH	Smoking cessation counseling Weight loss counseling Referral to sexual therapist Premarin 1.25 mg P.O. qD Provera 5 mg P.O. qD x 12 q mo	Decrease in smoking 5 lb weight loss Resolution of perimenopausal symptoms	3

Example 10 "Too Long" — The Right Way

#	Initials	Age	Gravida	Para	Problem	Diagnostic Procedures	Treatment	Results	No. of Visits
6	C.E.	26	5	1	Habitual aborter (first trimester)	Products of conception, karyotype (normal) Cervical cultures (normal) Hysterosalpingogram (normal) Immunologic evaluation initial screen: ANA (normal) APTT (normal) Anti-cardiolipin (minimally elevated) Lymphocytotoxic antibodies ordered Thyroid function tests (normal)	Referral to reproductive endocrinologist	Referral pending	4

Chapter 5 • The Case List

Example 11 "Too Short" — The Wrong Way

#	Initials & Hosp. No.	Age	Gravida	Para	Gest. Age	Complications Antepartum	Delivery or Postpartum	Operative Procedures and/ or Treatment	Days in Hosp.	Newborn Complications	Wgt.	Apgar 1 & 5 Minutes	Days in Hosp.
A.	Antepartum Admissions												
1	BG078331	24	3	2	34	Preterm labor	Undelivered	Intravenous tocolytics	2				
2	BJ026739	33	4	2	33	Preeclampsia, prior cesarean section	Undelivered	Aldomet, bedrest, transport to tertiary hospital	1				
3	BR026529	21	4	3	20	Pyelonephritis	Undelivered	Intravenous antibiotics	3				
4	GP009562	25	4	1	34	Preterm labor	Undelivered	Intravenous tocolytics					
5	JA066650	22	1	0	30	No prenatal care, preterm labor	Undelivered	Intravenous tocolytics, steroids, transport to tertiary hospital	0				
6	BM47315	27	4	3	16	13 cm right upper quadrant mass		Excision of dermoid cyst	2				

Example 12 "Too Short" — The Right Way

#	Initials & Hosp. No.	Age	Gravida	Para	Diagnosis Preoperative or Admission (include size of ovarian cysts)	Treatment	Surgical Pathology Diagnosis (uterine wt. in gms.)	Complications (include blood transfusions)	Days in Hosp.
29	L.P. 218515	32	3	2	Left labial tear	Repair of left labial tear		0	0

Chapter 5 • The Case List

Example 13 Too Many Patients Per Page

#	Initials	Age	Gravida	Para	Problem	Diagnostic Procedures	Treatment	Results	# Visits
Preventative Care & Health Maintenance									
174	RA	35	3	2012	Annual exam Polycystic ovaries	Pap, baseline mammogram Cardiac profile, fasting glucose	Dietary modification	Elevated cholesterol Glucose normal	1
175	AG	73	0	0	Annual exam Breast CA x 1 yr, on tamoxifen Atrophic vaginitis (pruritus)	Pap Endometrial biopsy: atrophic	Topical estrogen	Resolution of pruritus	3
Obesity									
Sexual Dysfunction									
176	ME	50	2	2004	Decreased libido on HRT	None	Testosterone added to HRT Testosterone increased	Slight improvement Significant improvement	6
Contraceptive Complications									
177	BB	31	0	0	Amenorrhea on birth control pills	Pregnancy test: negative	Changed formula	Regular menses	2
178	VM	63	5	5	Postmenopausal bleeding IUD perforating through cervix	IUD culture: actinomyces Endometrial biopsy: atrophic	PCN G 500 qd x 4 wk	No recurrent bleeding	6
Genetic Problems									
Primary or Secondary Amenorrhea									
179	JG	33	2	0010	48 days from last menses Requesting medical VIP	Pelvic sonogram (6-wk gestation) hCG, CBS, AST, ALT: normal	Methotrexate IM Misoprostol intravaginal	SAB	4
180	SO	27	0	0	Secondary amenorrhea Galactorrhea	Elevated prolactin (97) Pituitary MRI: microadenoma	Bromocriptine	Cyclic menses Galactorrhea improved	4
181	LW	25	0	0	Post-pill amenorrhea x 8 wk	Pregnancy test: negative TSH, prolactin: normal	Provera challenge	Menses	2
Infertility									
182	DB	32	1	1	Secondary infertility Irregular menses	TSH = hypothyroidism	Synthroid	Cyclic menses	2
183	JM	31	1	1	Secondary infertility	HSG: no abnormalities TSH, prolactin: normal Semen analysis: low sperm count	None	Referral: reproductive endocrinologist	3
Endometriosis									
184	AP	25	0	0	Severe dysmenorrhea History of endometriosis	None	Birth control pills Anaprox	Improvement	2

Example 14 Edited Version of Example 12

#	Initials	Age	Gravida	Para	Problem	Diagnostic Procedures	Treatment	Results	# Visits
1. Patient List
Preventative Care & Health Maintenance
153	RA	35	3	2	Annual exam Polycystic ovary disease	Pap, baseline mammogram Cardiac profile, 2h glucose test	Dietary modification	Elevated cholesterol Glucose normal	2
154	AG	73	0	0	Annual exam Breast cancer x 1 yr, on tamoxifen Atrophic vaginitis (pruritus)	Pap Endometrial biopsy: atrophic	Topical estrogen (discussed with breast surgeon and oncologist)	Resolution of atrophy	3
Obesity -None Observed
Sexual Dysfunction
155	ME	50	2	4	Decreased libido on HRT	None	Testosterone added to HRT	Improvement	6
Contraceptive Complicactions
156	BB	31	0	0	Amenorrhea on oral contraceptives	Pregnancy test: negative	Changed Estrogen from 20 mg to 30 mg	Regular menses	2
157	VM	63	5	5	Postmenopausal bleeding IUD perforating through cervix	IUD culture: actinomycoses Endometrial biopsy: atrophic	IUD removed PCN G 500 x qd 4 wk	No recurrence	6
Genetic Problems

Chapter 5 • The Case List

Patient Name   *Date*

Example 15   Shadows, Fonts

#	Initials	Age	Gravida	Para	Problem	Diagnostic Procedures	Treatment	Results	No of Visits
1. Patient List									
Preventative Care & Health Maintenance									
153	RA	35	3	2	Annual Exam Polycystic Ovary Disease	Pap, Baseline Mammogram Lipid Profile, 2h Glucose Test	Dietary Modification	Elevated cholesterol Glucose Normal	2
154	AG	73	0	0	Annual Exam Breast Cancer x 1 yr on Tamoxifen Vaginal pruritis	Pap Endometrial Biopsy: atrophic	Topical Estrogen (discussed w/Breast Surgeon & Oncologist)	Resolution	3
Obesity									
Sexual Dysfunction									
155	ME	50	2	4	Decreased libido on HRT	None	Testosterone added to HRT	Improvement	6

89

Example 16 Spaces for Organization

Candidate's Name:
Caselist Number:

LIST OF GYNECOLOGICAL PATIENTS *Post Residency Cases

July 1, 2009 - June 30, 2010
Page 11

#	HOSP #	Pat #	Age	GRAV	PARA	Diagnosis: Preoperative or Admission (Include size of ovarian cysts)	Treatment	Surgical Pathology Diagnosis (Uterine weight in gms.)	Complications (Include blood transfusions)	Days in Hosp
30	B	B-3	38	3	2	HMB Unsuccessful hormonal management Declined levonorgestral IUD and Ablation Genuine Stress Urinary Incontinence No uterine decensus	TLH TOT, Cystoscopy	Uterus - 129 gms - Adenomyosis Cervix - benign	None	1

Chapter 5 • The Case List

Example 17 Demarcating Lines

Candidate's Name:
Hospital Name:

LIST OF GYNECOLOGICAL PATIENTS

July 1, 2009 - June 30, 2010
Page 6

#	Initials & Hosp #	Age	GRAV	PARA	Diagnosis: Preoperative or Admission (Include size of ovarian cysts)	Treatment	Surgical Pathology Diagnosis (Uterine weight in grams)	Complications (Include blood transfusions)	Days in Hosp
23	D.H.	44	4	4	~HMB	~TAH - BS&O	~Uterine Wt. - 184 gms	None	2
	601512				~Pelvic Pain		~Adenomyosis		
					~Right Adrenal Mass : 6 x 7cm		~Right Ovary: Papillary serous Cyst Adenoma		
							~Left Ovary: Benign		

Example 18 Bulleted Items

LIST OF OBSTETRICAL PATIENTS

Name:

All Cases are Post Residency
Page 4

CA SE #	HOSP # PAT #	Age	Gravida	Para	Complications		Operative Procedure and/or Treatments	Days in Hosp	NEWBORN			
					Antepartum	Delivery or Postpartum			Perinatal Death	Wt.	Apgars 1 & 5 Mins	Days in Hosp
Preterm Delivery												
16	A15	25	1	0	• Preterm Contractions @ 25 weeks	• Preterm Delivery ○ Maternal exhaustion	• FFN- (Neg) ○ Cervical Length 3-4cm ○ Nifedipine • Spontaneous labor ○ Low forceps	2	N	2380	8 9	2

Example 19 Capital Letters   Emphasis & Abbreviations

LIST OF GYNECOLOGICAL PATIENTS   *Post Residency Cases

Candidate's Name:
Caselist Number

July 1, 2009 - June 30, 2010
Page 6

#	HOSP #	PAT #	AGE	GRAV	PARA	DIAGNOSIS: PREOPERATIVE OR ADMISSION (Include size of ovarian cysts)	TREATMENT	SURGICAL PATHOLOGY DIAGNOSIS (Uterine weight in gms.)	COMPLICATIONS (Include blood transfusions)	DAYS IN HOSP
ECTOPIC PREGNANCY										
12	A	A-9	36	2	0	Ruptured LEFT ectopic pregnancy H/O salpingostomy for RIGHT ectopic pregnancy Hemodynamically stable	Laparoscopic left salpingectomy	Fallopian tube with degenerated chorionic villi.	None	1

Example 20   Underline, Italicize, Bold

Name:

LIST OF OBSTETRICAL PATIENTS

All Cases are Post Residency
Page 26

CASE #	HOSP # PAT #	Age	GRAV	PARA	Complications - Antepartum	Complications - Delivery or Postpartum	Operative Procedure and/or Treatments	Days in Hosp	NEWBORN - Perinatal Death	NEWBORN - Wt.	NEWBORN - Apgars 1 & 5 Mins	NEWBORN - Days in Hosp
Trauma in Pregnancy (automobile accidents)												
177	A174	23	1	0	• Twin pregnancy • Automobile accident @ _**18**_ wks • Spontaneous labor ○ Declined attempted vaginal delivery	None	• Routine Growth Surveillance • Primary CD	3	N N	2353 2380	9 9 9 9	2 3
Pregnancies and coexisting malignancies												
178	A175	26	1	0	<u>Malignant Melanoma</u> @37 wks	• Meconium	• Wide local excision of melanoma & sentinel node- (Neg) • Cytotec induction ○ low forceps	2	N	3444	5 8	2

94

Chapter 5 • The Case List

Example 21   Bold

LIST OF OBSTETRICAL PATIENTS   *Post Residency Cases

Candidate's Name:
Case list ID # 612079

July 1, 2009 – June 30, 2010
Page | 18

#	HOSP #	Pa I #	AGE	GRAV	PARA	GEST AGE	ANTEPARTUM	COMPLICATIONS DELIVERY OR POSTPARTUM	OPERATIVE PROCEDURES AND OR TREATMENT	DAYS IN HOSP	PERI NATAL DEATH	NEWBORN WGT gms	APGAR 1/5 MIN	DAYS IN HOSP
REPEAT CESAREAN DELIVERY														
61	A	A-61	34	6	5	38	**Previous CD x 5** Limited Prenatal Care Presented in Labor Prolonged Bradycardia **Suspected uterine rupture** Desires sterilization		Stat Repeat CD Bilateral Tubal Ligation	3	N	1842	5/8	12

95

Example 22 Shading Every Other Line

Candidate's Name:
Caselist Number: 1

July 1, 2011–June 30, 2012
Page 1

Summary Sheet: All hospitals combined

Office Practice:

I. Office Practice Categories	Total cases	Total Applied
Preventive care and health maintenance	2	2
Contraception	2	2
Primary and secondary amenorrhea and hirsutism	2	2
Perimenopause and menopausal care	2	2
Office Surgery	2	2
Abnormal Uterine Bleeding	2	1
Evaluation and management of pelvic pain	2	2
Vaginal discharge	2	2
Vulvar disease	1	1
Breast Diseases	2	2
Evaluation of Urinary and Rectal Incontinence	2	2
Urinary tract infections	2	2
Sexually transmitted diseases	2	2
Immunizations	2	2
Dysmenorrhea	2	2
Premenstrual Syndrome	2	2
Benign Pelvic Masses	2	2
Ultrasound	2	2
Pelvic floor defects	2	2
Non-surgical office procedures (IUD insertion)	2	2
Preconception counseling	2	2
Total cases	40	40

II. Total number of ultrasound and Color Doppler Examinations in:
    A. Obstetrical patients: 70
    B. Gynecological patients: 10
    C. Other areas such as abdominal, thoracic, pediatric, etc.: 0

Example 23 Appropriate Friedman Terminology

#	Initials & Hosp. No.	Age	Gravida	Para	Gest. Age	Complications			Operative Procedures and/or Treatment	Days in Hosp.	Newborn			
						Antepartum	Delivery or Postpartum				Complications	Wgt.	Apgar 1 & 5 Minutes	Days in Hosp.
127	M.D. 175600	27	2	0	42	Post dates Protracted active phase of dilatation	Persistent occiput posterior position Arrest of descent		Cytotec cervical ripening Intrauterine pressure catheter Pitocin augmentation Failed low vacuum extraction Primary low transverse cesarean section	4	None	3686	9/10	4

Example 24 Management Flow — The Wrong Way

#	Initials & Hosp. No.	Age	Gravida	Para	Gest. Age	Complications		Operative Procedures and/or Treatment	Days in Hosp.	Newborn				
						Antepartum	Delivery or Postpartum			Complications	Wgt.	Apgar 1 & 5 Minutes	Days in Hosp.	
11	PH001118	37	1	0	36	Advanced maternal age, preterm, premature rupture of membranes, pregnancy-induced hypertension, Hypothyroidism	None	Synthroid, labetalol, Pitocin augmentation, low forceps delivery	3	None	3156	7/8	3

Chapter 5 • The Case List

Example 25 Management Flow — The Right Way

Initials & Hosp. # No.	Age	Gravida	Para	Diagnosis Preoperative or Admission (include size of ovarian cysts)	Treatment	Surgical Pathology Diagnosis (uterine wt. in gms.)	Complications (include blood transfusions)	Days in Hosp.
62 P.C. 372236	45	2	2	Abnormal uterine bleeding Endometrial thickening by vaginal sonography: 2.1 cm Stenotic cervix Office endometrial biopsy—unsuccessful	D&C	Endometrium- Dyssynchronous	None	0

Example 26 Pertinent Data "Just Right"

#	Initials & Hosp. No.	Age	Gravida	Para	Gest. Age	Complications		Operative Procedures and/or Treatment	Days in Hosp.	Newborn				
						Antepartum	Delivery or Postpartum			Complications	Wgt.	Apgar 1 & 5 Minutes	Days in Hosp.	
124	L.V. 100489	30	2	1	38	None	Severe shoulder dystocia	Spontaneous vaginal delivery McRobert's maneuver, Suprapubic pressure, Episiotomy extension (third degree) Wood's corkscrew maneuver	2	None	3912	8/9	2	

Chapter 6

Kodachromes

The Kodachrome section was ELIMINATED in 2003. For those of the digital generation, Kodachromes are 35-mm slides that are projected images. A few isolated ones have surfaced since 2003 and they are now projected onto the laptop screen. They may represent any Ob/Gyn topic, but their role on the exam has shifted. Initially, the emphasis was on correct identification of the slide. Later, they were used as a starting point for discussion of a particular topic and comprised no more than 25% of the exam.

Historically, there were six to nine slides: two or three each for obstetrics, gynecology, and office practice. The set of slides changed daily. Typically, the slides were labeled with the diagnosis; although usually at least one diagnosis was unknown.

Obviously, the labeled slides stated the diagnosis up front. Although correct identification of the unknown slide scored points, you did not lose points if you did not identify the slide correctly.

The examiners recognized that the unlabeled slides were subject to interpretation.

Thus, there may have been more than one correct answer for each slide. The emphasis was not on your correct identification of the Kodachrome, but on the justification for your interpretation. Variable interpretations were a springboard for a variety of topics. The examiner had less control of the agenda and you then had the opportunity for expression of individual, creative thinking and spontaneous discussion of various topics. On the other hand, a labeled slide set a defined agenda and allowed standardization among candidates.

If you can picture a topic, it can easily be projected. The ACOG on line CREOG QUIZ is a good reference since the questions always start with a picture. The difference is that they are followed by written questions, so all you need to do is turn them into an oral discussion. You can also turn many of the structured cases into a kodachrome or image.

Let me help you get started. For whatever you are visualizing, ask yourself the following questions:
>   What does this image portray?
>   What are the clinical implications?
>   How would you work it up?
>   What is your differential diagnosis?
>   How would you manage the patient?
>   What are potential complications?

Obstetrics is the easiest since we deal with ultrasound images daily. What are some logical questions with an ultrasound image?

> What does this image portray?
>> Fetus
>>> How many?
>>>> Any abnormalities? If so, what are the characteristic ultrasound features? Describe features for Trisomy 16, 18, 21, Turner's etc
>>> Position
>>> Growth abnormalities: IUGR, macrosomia
>> Placenta
>>> Location
>>> Features
>>> Cord insertion
>> Amniotic fluid
>>> Oligo vs. polyhydramnios
>>> Infection
>>>> Fetal heart rate tracings are an obvious picture too
>>>>> Interpretation
>>>>> Category
>>>>> Management
>>>>> Non-stress tests
>>>>> OCTs
>>> OB Emergencies
>>>> Malpresentation: Breech, Transverse lie, Mentum, Brow
>>>> Abruption
>>>> Cord prolapsed
>>>> Shoulder dystocia
>>>> Postpartum hemorrhage
>>>> Uterine inversion
>>> Genetics
>>>> Family tree and interpretation of inheritance pattern eg-autosomal recessive, dominant, X-linked recessive, translocation
>>> Follow up discussion on each inheritable disease

Chapter 6 • Kodachromes

Gynecology pictures are not as intuitive as Obstetrics, but if you start thinking about it, you can come up with all kinds of possibilities. The OR is a logical place to start, since those are pictures that we also see daily.

- Hysterectomy – think of any conceivable twist
  - Pre op
    - Fibroids
  - Intra op
    - Challenges, complications, imaging
      - Adhesions
      - Bowel injury
      - Bladder injury
  - Post op
    - Cuff dehiscence
  - Route
- Incisions
  - Types
  - Complications
    - Infection
    - Dehiscence
- Laparoscopy
  - Set up
  - Equipment
  - Trocar placement and mishaps
    - Vessel injury
    - Visceral injury
- Emergencies
  - Ectopic pregnancy
    - Work up
    - Location
    - Management
  - Ovarian torsion
- Female Pelvic Medicine
  - Prolapse and Urinary/Fecal incontinence
    - Work up
    - Surgical and non-surgical management
    - Complications
- Oncology
  - Each organ system depicting the cancer, work up, management, complications
  - Microscopic slides
  - Colposcopy: features delineating benign, dysplasia, cancer
- Ultrasound
  - Ovarian masses: features delineating benign vs malignant
  - Uterus: Fibroids, endometrial stripe, sonohysterogram

Office, like GYN, necessitates having to think outside the box. However, the possibilities are endless.

STDs
    Gross (literally) & microbiology pictures of each one, then differential diagnosis, work up, management

Vaginitis
    Gross (literally), microscopic, & microbiology appearance for each one

Vulvar
    Gross and microscopic: LSA, Vulvar dystrophy, Bechet's, Paget's, funny looking moles

Pediatric
    Labial agglutination
    How to examine
    Foreign body
    Straddle injury

Sexual assault

REI
    Ultrasound
        PCOS
        Mullerian abnormalities
        Funny looking people with characteristic congenital abnormalities: Turner's, Klinefelter's, ambiguous genitalia, 5-alpha reductase deficiency
    Infertility
        Ultrasound and imaging of congenital abnormalities
    PCOS
        Hirsutism, acanthosis nigracans, ultrasound PCOS
    Endometriosis
    Intraoperative photos

In conclusion, since images were deleted in 2003, don't waste a lot of time speculating about what might reappear if reintroduced. However, this exercise is helpful to get you to think outside the box, which will only help to deepen your depth, breadth and ultimate mastery of a topic.

Chapter 7

Case of the Day

"Case of the Day" is my term for what the board refers to as Structured and/or Simulated Cases. The case of the day was introduced in 1994 when they replaced the pathology microscopic slides interpretation; half of the exam entailed the kodachromes and the other half was the case of the day. This change signaled the board's attempt to standardize the exam and introduce more objectivity to an inherently subjective format.

The purpose of the structured cases, per the ABOG *Bulletin*, is to interpret a candidate's response to specific clinical situations. Typically, each case starts with a written patient management scenario that is projected onto a screen and serves as a springboard for a specific topic. Standardized follow up questions ensue. Unlike the questions during the case list section of the exam, ABOG (not the examiner) predetermines most of these questions.

All candidates being examined on the same day have the same structured cases; hence, my nickname "case of the day". There is a different set of cases every day. In 2003, when the kodachromes were deleted, the exam was limited to defending your case list and the case of the day. Therefore, half of your test, or 30 minutes, is devoted to the case of the day.

Like other exam components, the case of the day has also evolved. Over the years, the number of cases fluctuated from a minimum of three to as many as seven. Like Goldilocks, ABOG decided the "just right" number was five. Each section starts with the case of the day, and then switches to defending your case list for the last half.

Since the questions are predetermined and everyone is asked the same questions, the answers are predictable. As with any test, there is a bell-shaped curve of expected answers and the board has set a threshold of knowledge that must be reached to pass the topic. The format of the case of the day dictates standardization, yet the oral exam component permits flexibility to go beyond the threshold or to pursue other topics.

Typically, the topic is a common management issue that the generalist frequently faces. Therefore, the topics on your case list probably overlap with these topics, so you will already be prepared. The questions require you to manage the patient systematically and to progress down the algorithm pathway, as you do every day in your practice. One of the five topics may be less common, but take comfort that your cohorts answering the same questions will share the same level of unfamiliarity.

The examiners don't even get to see the case of the day questions until the morning of the test, at which time they collectively discuss the answers. Sometimes they don't even agree among themselves as to the correct answer. Rarely, even the examiners won't know the answers to some of the obscure and difficult questions. The examiners are provided guidelines by ABOG, but are given latitude as to how to extract and interpret your answers, as well as the freedom to supplement with their own questions. Although only one of the pair of examiners is questioning you, both must be in agreement regarding your resulting score.

The strategy for the case of the day session is straightforward. There are five sets of cases lasting a total of 30 minutes. Thus, you should spend no longer than six minutes for each set. In 2008, the chime to signal the halfway point at 30 minutes and to cue the switch to the case list was eliminated. You don't need to worry about the time, as it is the examiner's responsibility to keep you on pace. Nonetheless, you don't want to dilly-dally on this session. The more questions you answer, the more points you score, and the more you dilute the wrong answers. It is not necessary to, and rarely do you, get all answers correct. Although ABOG does not reveal their grading scale, logically you probably just need to get the majority (at least 70%) correct to pass each set. So if there are five cases, you can miss one set and score an overall pass for 4/5 or 80%. However, you cannot fail two sets, as 3/5 is only 60% and will most likely result in an overall fail.

Practice is paramount to assure your success. The case of the day is clearly an example of "don't let them see you sweat". Often times, the answer to the previous question is revealed in the next cued question. Don't be rattled if you chose a different answer. Remember, you don't have to get every question correct—just the majority. So use this as an opportunity to get back on track. Don't compromise the whole set by getting unglued by one question. Besides, even if your answer is different, this doesn't necessarily mean you missed the question. Don't forget that most the time, there is more than one way to "skin a cat", especially in medicine.

For example, let's say the question asked is "How would you treat a patient with endometrial hyperplasia with atypia?" Let's say you chose a hysteroscopic-guided fractional D&C. But the next cued question starts out, "The patient is treated with progesterone and …". Was your answer of D&C correct? Of course, but the test writer has to move the question along and elected to go down the left, rather than your right, fork of the patient management algorithm pathway. So don't get frustrated and blow the rest of the questions. Switch gears, go with the flow, recover and concentrate fully on this next question with the new information.

The case of the day is typically one of two formats. The first is management of a specific patient from beginning to end. The other is a theme that they spin and turn. For example, the theme may be abnormal uterine bleeding in an adolescent, then in a reproductive aged woman and then in a postmenopausal woman.

The case of the day is typically fair and straightforward. These are not trick questions. The question is right there in black and white on the computer screen. Don't make the questions harder than they are. Chances are, if you're stumped, so are your colleagues.

However, unlike on your case list, try to avoid replying that you don't know the answer to a question. The examiner will have no choice but to completely dock all the points for that sub-question. So if you guess, or at least think out loud, hopefully you can get partial credit. The worse thing that can happen is that you don't get any credit. Remember also, that out of your group, somebody is most likely going to know the answer. Again, you have nothing to lose; or rather you have everything to gain, by trying to score as many points as possible.

Just a couple of practice sessions are all that is necessary to get the hang of it. The trick is finding a review course or products that can simulate this aspect of the exam. Because this section of the exam is on the computer, there is a tendency to fixate and talk into the computer screen, rather than replying directly to the examiner. Initially, an awkward dilemma arises as to who and if the question should be read aloud. Go with the examiner's cue. Some will read the question out loud to you and others will ask you to reply when ready. If you are so nervous and have

ADD tendencies that are distracting your attention with subconscious trash talk, read the question out loud. If on the other hand, you can concentrate better by reading silently, respond when you are ready.

Pen and paper are available to take notes. Do NOT write out a treatise before you answer out loud. This will waste precious time. It would be OK to jot down some quick notes if it facilitates your answer. For example, if the question is, "What's your differential diagnosis for abnormal uterine bleeding?", you might write PALM-COEIN as a mnemonic prompter.

Although any topic is fair game, the Foundation for Exxcellence in Women's Health, sponsored in part by ABOG, has published a monthly review of the most challenging topics on the oral exam since 2008. This list can be found in *The Pearls of Exxcellence*, accessible by http://www.exxcellence.org/pearls.php. Since these were determined to be challenging exam topics, they most likely came from the cases of the day. In Table 1, I have listed *The Pearls of Exxcellence* topics since their origin.

Another obvious source of case of the day topics could be from your case list categories. You're accountable for these topics even if you didn't choose a representative patient, so you must know them anyway.

When preparing your oral defense for the case of the day, ask yourself the same questions you do when proceeding down the patient management algorithm pathway. The three questions that summarize the approach are:

>What is your differential diagnosis?
>
>How would you work her up?
>
>What is your management?

As you answer each question, try to brainstorm all possible permutations. I'll walk through some possibilities with each of the above main questions, but I think you'll agree that the possibilities are endless. Thus, your preparation can easily extend beyond the six minutes that are allotted for each case.

In answering the question, "What is your differential diagnosis?", you want to show a deep depth and breadth with your response. Also, your response directly impacts the answers to the subsequent questions. If you can come up with only 3-5 possibilities, your subsequent work up is entirely dependent upon your working diagnoses. To assure the necessary depth and breadth, describe the forest before the trees. A reasonable starting point for any differential diagnosis is to categorize them into gynecologic and non-gynecologic causes. Next, divide either track by organ system.

Non-gynecologic causes may include psychosomatic, musculoskeletal, gastrointestinal, urologic, etc. Likewise, gynecologic causes include ovarian, uterine, fallopian tube, cervical, vaginal and vulvar. You could also include infectious, pregnancy, benign or malignant causes.

I think you get the idea. Just keep drilling down further and further. Be organized, methodical and succinct. Don't just randomly blurt out diagnoses in no particular order. This might be a good time to jot some quick notes before you answer, but only if you think it will organize your thoughts and facilitate your reply without wasting precious time.

This is especially important when answering the question, "How would you work her up?". You want to show that you are resourceful and thoughtful with your resources. For your laboratory evaluation, start first with initial labs and reserve ordering other labs until you have interpreted the initial results. Likewise for imaging studies - order the logical and ideally most cost prudent studies first and then order exotic and expensive studies only if necessary.

I hope you can see that how well you answered the first two questions directly impacts your management. This reflects your ability to hone in on the diagnosis after weeding others out based upon the results of your work up. However, once you decide on the most likely diagnosis, you again want to be resourceful and thoughtful with your management. Ideally, you would again start conservatively and resort to surgery lastly.

Conservative measures include a list of options, which may include physical or psychotherapy, expectant or medications. Pharmacologic options should also incorporate the forest and tree analogy. Describe first the classes of drugs, eg. hormonal, NSAIDs, anti-fibrinolytics, etc. Now describe sub-classes if appropriate, eg. progestins, estrogens, GnRH agonists, etc. for hormones. Can you drill down even further? eg. OCPs (COC —cyclic or continuous, Progestin-only), Mirena, Nexplanon. DMPA, etc. for progestins.

Another top-to-bottom approach in preparing for a topic is to approach it with my "no stones unturned" concept. This is tedious, but exhaustive and comprehensive and it approaches a topic from all angles.

For any topic, see if you can answer the following questions:

> Can this topic be defined? eg. endometriosis
>
> Are there any epidemiologic issues? eg. incidence, prevalence, positive/negative predictive value (eg. quadruple maternal serum screening)

What is the pathogenesis or etiology? (eg. endometriosis)

How do you make the diagnosis?

Diagnosis of exclusion

Laboratory evaluation

Imaging

Biopsy

What is the treatment?

Conservative

Medical

Surgical

What is the expected outcome of each treatment? (eg. PCOS, cancer)

What is the appropriate follow up? (eg. cancer surveillance)

Finally, remember they can approach a question from any order in the algorithm pathway. Don't expect them to always start at the beginning. The question is right there in black and white on the computer screen, so you can always orient yourself. Bottom line is to answer the question, directly and succinctly. Show that you are organized in your thought process and utilization of resources. Give the examiner a positive mental image of how you actually approach patients every day.

I suggest you walk through each of the *Pearls* as well as the case list categories and ask yourself the above three questions. Better yet, have a colleague quiz you and see how many different pathways can stem from each question. If you keep drilling down, I guarantee you'll eventually strike oil and come up with a pass!

TABLE 7.1 Pearls of Exxcellence Topics (since 2008)

GYNECOLOGY

ECTOPIC PREGNANCY
1. Diagnosis and Management of Ectopic Pregnancy (January 2014)

GI TRACT INJURIES
1. Management of Postoperative Ileus (March 2010, revised December 2015)
2. Incidental Enterotomy – Small Bowel Injury (December 2010)
3. Large Bowel Injury – Simple (December 2010)

HYSTERECTOMY
1. Management of a Lost Pedicle at the time of a Vaginal Hysterectomy (February 2013)
2. Management of Evisceration of the Vaginal Cuff (May 2014)
3. Surgery in Morbidly Obese Patients (September 2014)

HYSTEROSCOPY
1. Management of Lateral Uterine Perforations at Time of Hysteroscopy (July 2012)
2. Perforation with Uterine Sound and Suction Cannula during a D&C (March 2014)
3. Postmenopausal bleeding in a woman with a Stenotic Cervix (December 2015)

INFECTION
1. Sepsis (December 2015)

LAPAROSCOPIC COMPLICATIONS
1. Complications of Gynecologic Laparoscopic Surgery (May 2015, replaces September 2009)
2. Avoiding Trocar Injuries Associated with Laparoscopic Surgery (February 2012)

THROMBOEMBOLISM
1. Perioperative Management of Anticoagulation in Gynecologic Patients (January 2011 revised December 2015)
2. Evaluation of Dyspnea and Management of Pulmonary Embolism After Surgery (November 2014)
3. Management of Women on Hormonal Therapy or Contraception in Women Undergoing Surgery (September 2015)

OBSTETRICS

ADNEXAL MASS
1. Pregnant Women with an Adnexal Mass (September 2015, replaces June 2009) by Management of Adnexal Masses in Pregnancy

ALLOIMMUNIZATION
1. Nonimmune Hydrops Fetalis (January 2009)
2. Management of Pregnancy with ABO Incompatibility (September 2011)
3. Cytomegalovirus Infection in Pregnancy (September 2013)

AMNIOTIC FLUID EMBOLISM
1. Amniotic Fluid Embolism (April 2013)

CEREBRAL PALSY
1. Cerebral Palsy (July 2009)
2. Neonatal Encephalopathy (July 2010)

CESAREAN DELIVERY
1. Management of Broad Ligament Extension and Hematoma during a Cesarean Delivery (May 2013)
2. Management of Wound Complications of Cesarean Delivery (July 2014)
3. Intrapartum and Postpartum Fever (June 2014)

DIABETES
1. Pre-gestational Diabetes Diagnosed in Early Pregnancy (June 2015)

FETAL ANOMALIES
1. Fetal Ventral Abdominal Wall Defects (January 2015, replaces March 2009)

FETAL MONITORING
1. Fetal Heart Rate Abnormalities: Minimal Variability and Heart Rate of 100 (March 2014)

HYPERTENSIVE DISORDERS OF PREGNANCY
1. Postpartum Eclampsia (November 2015)

INFECTIONS IN PREGNANCY
1. Fetal Infections – Parvo, CMV, Toxo (October 2008)
2. Maternal and Fetal Complications of Varicella at Term (September 2012)
3. Cytomegalovirus Infection in Pregnancy (September 2013)
4. Intrapartum and Postpartum Fever (June 2014)
5. Trichomonas, Gonorrhea, and Chlamydia in Pregnancy (November 2015)
6. Sepsis (December 2015)

MALPRESENTATION
1. Management of Malpresentations: brow, face and compound (December 2011)
2. Management of the Frank Breech Presenting at the Introitus (December 2013)

MEDICAL COMPLICATIONS OF PREGNANCY

HEMATOLOGIC DISORDERS
1. Anemia in Pregnancy with Normal Iron Studies (April 2010)
2. Evaluation of Anemia in Pregnancy

PLACENTA
1. Placentomegaly (November 2010)
2. Etiology and Management of Placenta Accreta at 20 Weeks (July 2011)
3. Etiology and Management of Vasa Previa (October 2011)

PRENATAL RISK MANAGEMENT
1. Elevated Maternal Serum AFP at 16 Weeks (June 2010)

TRAUMA IN PREGNANCY
1. Postpartum Perineal Pain (October 2009)

Chapter 7 • Case of the Day

TWINS
1. Management of Twins (March 2012)
2. Management of Multi-fetal Pregnancy: monochorionic, diamnioninc twins; monochorionic, monoamnionic twins (November 2012)

OFFICE EXAM

ADOLESCENT GYNECOLOGY
1. Adnexal Masses in Adolescents (April 2015, replaces May 2009)

CONTRACEPTION
1. Women on Oral Contraceptives (November 2008)
2. Contraceptive Choices for Women with Common Medical Problems (August 2010)
3. Essure in Place, Now Desires Pregnancy (August 2011)
4. Management of Women on Hormonal Therapy or Contraception in Women Undergoing Surgery (September 2015)
5. Contraception in Women with Cardiovascular Risk Factors (September 2015)
6. Hormonal Contraception in Women Taking Medications with Potential Drug Interactions (October 2015)
7. Contraception in Women with Lupus (October 2015)
8. Contraception in Women with Thromboembolism and Thrombophilia (October 2015)

DOMESTIC VIOLENCE
1. Management of a Patient Who Has Suffered Domestic Violence (January 2015)

DYSLIPIDEMIA
1. Dyslipidemia and Metabolic Syndrome in Women (November 2009)

MENOPAUSE
1. Postmenopausal Ovarian Mass (March 2009)
2. Risks of Hormone Therapy (November 2011)
3. Evaluation of Postmenopausal Bleeding (August 2014)
4. Management of Women on Hormonal Therapy or Contraception in Women Undergoing Surgery (September 2015)
5. Postmenopausal bleeding in a woman with a Stenotic Cervix (December 2015)

PID (PELVIC INFLAMMATORY DISEASE)
1. Management of Bilateral Tubo-Ovarian Abscesses in Young Nulligravida (March 2013)

SEXUALLY TRANSMITTED INFECTIONS
1. Management of Primary and Recurrent HSV 2 Vulvar Infections (November 2015)

THYROID DISEASE
1. Management of a Thyroid Nodule (January 2010)
2. Etiology and Management of Hypothyroidism (May 2011)

VAGINITIS
1. Management of Persistent and Recurrent Trichomonas (September 2015)

ONCOLOGY

ABNORMAL PAP SMEARS
1. Atypical Glandular Cells (January 2013)

BREAST CANCER
1. Ongoing Care of a Woman with Breast Cancer on Letrozole (June 2013)
2. Cystic Breast Masses in Young Women (August 2015)

OVARIAN CANCER
1. Pregnant Women with an Adnexal Mass (June 2009)
2. Adnexal Masses in Adolescents (May 2009)
3. Postmenopausal Ovarian Mass (March 2009)
4. Management of Adnexal Mass (October 2010)
5. Management of Adnexal Cysts (September 2010)

UTERINE CANCER
1. Surgical Management of the Obese Patient with Endometrial Cancer (December 2008)
2. Management When a Hysteroscopic or D&C Biopsy is Reported as a Grade I AC of the Endometrium (October 2014)

VAGINA
1. Management of Vaginal Cysts (June 2010)

VULVAR CANCER
1. Postmenopausal Vulvar Lesions (April 2009)
2. Management of Paget's Disease of the Vulva (May 2015, Replaces May 2010)

VULVAR BENIGN DERMATOLOGY
1. Postmenopausal Vulvar Lesions (April 2009)

REPRODUCTIVE ENDOCRINOLOGY & INFERTILITY (REI)

AMENORRHEA
1. Primary Amenorrhea in a Teenager (March 2011)

ENDOMETRIOSIS
1. Surgical Management of Endometriosis (January 2012)

HYPERPROLACTINEMIA
1. Hyperprolactinemia (April 2012)

INFERTILITY
1. Proximal Tubal Occlusion (November 2013)
2. Management of Women with Multiple Fibroids Who are Attempting Pregnancy (April 2014)

FEMALE PELVIC MEDICINE & RECONSTRUCTIVE SURGERY (FPMRS)

DIVERTICULA
 1. Management of Urethral Diverticula (February 2011)

EPISIOTOMY COMPLICATIONS
 1. Management of Breakdown of a 4th Degree Perineal Laceration (October 2012)
 2. Evaluation and Management of a 4th Degree Laceration (December 2014)
 3. Postpartum Perineal Pain (March 2015)

INCONTINENCE
 1. Complications of TVT (April 2011)
 2. Fecal Incontinence (February 2010)
 3. Voiding Dysfunction in TVT Patients (August 2012)

URETER
 1. Management of Ureteral Injuries (June 2011)

VAGINAL/VULVAR HEMATOMA
 1. Hematoma after a Vacuum Delivery (December 2012)

Chapter 8

Studying for the Exam

The focus of this book until now has been the individualized study strategy applied to specific phases of preparation for the oral exam. This chapter summarizes the process of studying in general.

You must first prioritize your study topics. Ideally, this is accomplished about six months before the exam, when you attend your first review course. Your objective in prioritizing is to identify and rank your personal strengths and weaknesses across the range of study topics that are covered during the review course.

Compare this list with topics that you know will be on the exam; namely, those exam topics that are published in the *Bulletin* and those on your case list. Finally, identify those topics that have been high yield during morning report throughout your residency, M&M conferences, and CREOG in-service training exams. Predictably, certain topics rise to the top. Those topics that I feel are the highest yield are called "Know Cold" topics in Table 1. Those topics that are important to know, but of lesser importance, I refer to as "Hot Topics" in Table 2. Each topic is followed by a line of questioning to answer during your review. The intent is not to be all-inclusive, but rather to stimulate you to ask even more probing questions.

Combine the above lists and draft an updated priority list. Stash it away for later reference. Next, funnel all your energy into compiling the case list. After the case list is cast in stone, identify the study topics that it generates. Cross-reference this study list with the earlier list generated above. Once again, compare the two lists and prioritize an updated list.

Dedicate one month, typically at least two months before your exam, to learn your case list cold. You should cover the majority of topics generated by your case list. Shuffle the remaining topics into the deck drafted earlier, and once again reprioritize an updated study list. The remaining time is spent in whittling away at the list. Some additional topics may be generated by mock oral exams. With only one month to go, accept the fact that it is impossible to cover the entire list. Reprioritize the remaining topics every week.

Stop in-depth studying one week before the exam. Spend the last week simply reviewing this mass of information. Solidify your strengths.

Polish articulation of this knowledge with mock oral exams. Refer to the end of the chapter for specific guidelines on how to make the most of this critical study aid. For this exam, it is simply not good enough to be only book smart.

I've presented the "Know-Cold" topics in an oral exam format to emphasize how studying for an oral exam is different than studying for a written exam. However, for sake of expediency, I've presented the study focus for the "Hot Topics" in the traditional approach. I challenge you throughout your studying to begin and end each like an oral exam. The best tool you have is your mouth. Literally talk out loud as you study; that alone will condition you to hearing yourself talk, increasing your comfort in articulation, and appreciating how you must adapt your studying for an oral exam.

TABLE 8.1 "Know Cold" Topics

I. Obstetrics

Shoulder Dystocia
- What are risk factors?
- Would you induce labor?
- Would you offer a CD?
- What is your protocol upon recognition?
- Describe the maneuvers
    - Suprapubic pressure
    - McRobert's maneuver
    - Corkscrew maneuvers
        - Wood's
        - Rubin's
        - Delivery of posterior arm
        - Gaskin Hands/Knees
        - Zavanelli

- What are the sequalae of brachial nerve plexus injury?
    - Describe Duchenne's palsy
    - Describe Klumpke's palsy
- What is your management in subsequent pregnancy?

Malpresentation: Breech
- What are the different types of breech and the incidence of cord prolapse associated with each?
- What are risk factors for breech presentation?
- What is the incidence at term?
- How do you counsel a patient interested in a vaginal breech delivery?
- Who are candidates?
- When is a vaginal breech delivery contraindicated?
- How is a breech delivered vaginally?
- What is head entrapment and how to solve?
- How do you manage nuchal arms?
- How do you apply Piper forceps?
- How and where do you make Dhrussen's incisions?
- Who are candidates for external cephalic version (ECV)?
- When is an ECV contraindicated?
- How do you counsel a patient?
- At what gestation do you plan your ECV?
- What are your orders in anticipation of an ECV to L&D?
- Describe your technique.
- What is your success?
- What are complications?
- When is Rhogam indicated and why?
- For each of the below malpresentations: Who can deliver vaginally? If not, why?
    - Brow
    - Mentum
        - Anterior
        - Posterior
    - Transverse
        - Back up
        - Back down
    - Compound

Postpartum Hemorrhage
- What are risk factors?
- What pre-op measures can you take if you anticipate a PPH?
- Differential diagnoses of postpartum hemorrhage?
    - How does your differential change if it is early vs delayed PPH?

- Define primary and secondary causes of PPH and give examples of each.
    - How to manage?
    - What uterotonics can be used?
        - Dose/schedule?
        - Mechanisms of action?
        - Side effects
        - Contraindications?
- Discuss tamponade techniques available for postpartum hemorrhage.
    - When are these techniques appropriate?
- Discuss the role and technique for each of the following surgical managements:
    - Utero-ovarian ligament ligation
    - O'Leary O'Leary uterine artery ligation
    - B-Lynch
    - Hemostatic box/square suture
    - Hypogastric artery ligation
- When is Rhogam indicated and why?
    - How do you determine the dose?
    - What is the maximum dose that can be given in 24 hours?
    - For how long will the patient's antibody screen be + after Rhogam?
- When would you treat PPH with uterine artery embolization?

Hypertensive Disorders of Pregnancy
- For each, discuss the following:
    - How do you make the diagnosis?
    - How does the disease affect the fetus and mom?
    - How do you manage the mom:
        - Antepartum
        - Intrapartum
        - Postpartum
    - What is the recurrence?
- Define each of the following:
    - Chronic hypertension
    - Gestational hypertension
    - Preeclampsia
    - Eclampsia
    - Acute fatty liver syndrome
    - HELLP syndrome

Diabetes
- Discuss preconception counseling for pre-gestational diabetic
- How does the HbA1C correlate with birth defects?

Chapter 8 • Studying for the Exam

- Discuss malformations of fetus associated with maternal DM.
    - What is the most common?
    - What is pathognomonic?
- What are risk factors for gestational diabetes (GDM)?
- When do you screen for GDM?
    - When would you screen early?
- Discuss the role of each of the following screening tests:
    - 1 hour GTT
    - 3 hour GTT
    - HbA1C
- What is the risk of GDM to:
    - Mom
    - Fetus
- Define each White's classification:
    - A1:
    - A2:
    - B:
    - C:
    - D:
    - F:
    - R:
- Discuss diabetic diet
    - How do you calculate the kcals?
    - How do you instruct her re: fat/CHO/protein?
    - How long do you give dietary management?
    - What are the options if she fails dietary management?
- What is the role for oral hypoglycemic (OHG) agents?
    - Which OHG do you prescribe?
    - What are the mechanisms of action of the more commonly prescribed OHGs?
- How do you monitor a GDM?
    - What is the role of fasting blood glucose monitoring?
    - What is the role for postprandial blood glucose monitoring?
    - What is your antepartum surveillance?
    - When do you recommend insulin management?
        - How do you start insulin?
        - Which type of insulins do you prescribe?
        - How do you monitor a patient on insulin?
        - What is your goal?
- Discuss the pathophysiology of diabetic ketoacidosis (DKA).
    - How do you diagnose DKA?
    - How do you manage a patient in DKA?
- When should delivery be timed?

- What is macrosomia?
    - How to manage?
    - What are the sequelae?

II. Gynecology

Ureter
- Describe the path of the ureter from the kidney to the bladder.
- What are the signs and symptoms of ureteral injury?
- How and when is serum creatinine level useful?
- Name 3 most common sites of injury and describe how injury occurs at those sites.
- Compare ipsilateral to contralateral reanastomosis.
- Describe reverse nephropexy, Boari flap, and psoas hitch.
- Discuss how to evaluate & repair intra-op and post-op.
- How to manage if there is no urologist available?
- Why use a ureteral stent?

Hysterectomy
- What are alternatives to hysterectomy?
- How do you determine the route for hysterectomy?
- Who are ideal candidates for a:
    - vaginal hysterectomy (VH)
    - laparoscopic-assisted vaginal hysterectomy (LAVH)
    - total laparoscopic hysterectomy (TLH)
    - robotic-assisted hysterectomy
    - abdominal hysterectomy
- How do you counsel for a prophylactic BSO or opportunistic salpingectomy?
- Discuss the impact on sexual function and prolapse.
- What is the role of antibiotic prophylaxis?
- What is the role of cystoscopy?
- What is your management if cancer is found on a frozen section?
- For each of the following complications:
    - How would cuff dehiscence &/or evisceration present?
    - How would you work her up?
    - What is the treatment?
- What is your differential diagnosis for cuff granulation?
    - How/when would it present?
    - How would you work her up?
    - What is the treatment?
- How do you routinely support your cuff to prevent prolapse?

III. Office Practice

Adnexal Mass
- What is your differential diagnosis for each of the following age groups?
    - Childhood
    - Adolescence
    - Reproductive
    - Menopausal
- How would you work up each age group?
    - Childhood
    - Adolescence
    - Reproductive
    - Menopausal
- What, if any, tumor markers would you order for each age group and what tumors are they specific for?
    - Childhood
    - Adolescence
    - Reproductive
    - Menopausal
- What U/S features are suggestive of:
    - benign mass
    - malignant mass
- What gross/clinical features are suggestive of:
    - benign mass
    - malignant mass
- What is the significance of a mass with a gross finding &/or imaging characterized by the following:
    - cystic mass
    - solid mass
    - complex mass
- What is the role for observation vs intervention?
- If surgery, how to decide the route, specifically laparotomy vs if laparoscopic removal?
- What are the sequelae if a dermoid ruptures? How to treat?
- What if frozen section diagnosis is malignancy?
- Discuss how to perform staging.

Amenorrhea (Secondary)
- Define
- What initial labs should be ordered?
- How do you proceed if the initial labs (HCG, Prolactin, TSH) are normal?
- What is your differential diagnosis if she has a progestin withdrawal bleed?
    - How do you now proceed?
- Describe physical characteristics of patient with anovulatory amenorrhea.

- What is your differential diagnosis if she does not have a progestin withdrawal bleed?
    How do you now proceed?
- What is your differential diagnosis if the FSH is elevated?
    How to further work up the patient?
- How do you diagnose POF?
    What is the cause of POF?

Preventive Care and Health Maintenance per AGE Group
- Who should have an annual exam?
- What should the exam include?
- What is the recommended screening for breast cancer?
- When to begin mammography?
    How often?
- When to begin colon cancer screening?
    How?
    How often?
- What are the recommendations for Pap smear screening?
    When to start?
    Stop?
- When to test for thyroid function?
    How?
    How often?
- When to test for dyslipidemias?
    How?
- When to test for diabetes?
    How?
- When to test for osteoporosis?
    How?
- Know treatment options for all of the above.

Immunizations
- Which ones are recommended for:
    Adolescent
    Reproductive age group
    >65 years old
- Which ones are indicated in pregnancy and why?
- Which ones are contraindicated in pregnancy and why?
- Discuss tetanus.
    When should a booster be given?
    Is it safe in pregnancy?
- What is Tdap?
    For whom is it indicated?

- What is the influenza vaccination?
    - Who are candidates?
- How long should a patient wait before conception after immunization or vaccination?
- Discuss HPV immunization
    - What is the protocol?
    - How effective is it?

Contraception
- How do you counsel patient on the variety of methods?
- How do you start a patient on a method?
- Discuss the mechanisms of action (multiple sites).
- What are the non-contraceptive benefits of hormonal contraceptives?

Barrier Method
- Discuss how you counsel a patient on the correct use of:
    - Condoms
    - Diaphragm
    - Spermicide
    - Sponge
- What are the non-contraceptive benefits of barriers?

Depomedroxyprogesterone Acetate (DMPA)
- How do you counsel a patient?
- Who are candidates?
- What is the mechanism of action?
- What is the FDA black box warning?
- How do you manage break through bleeding?
- What are the non-contraceptive benefits of DMPA?

Nexplanon
- What are the LARCs (long-acting reversible contraceptives) and compare them in terms of mechanism of action, length of use, side effects, and contraindications.
- How do you counsel a nulliparous adolescent who seeks your advice on LARCs?
- Discuss immediate postpartum insertion of LARCs.
- Discuss post-abortion insertion of LARCs.
- Discuss LARCs and emergency contraception.
    - How do you counsel a patient?
    - Who are candidates?
- What is the mechanism of action of Nexplanon?
    - Describe your insertion technique
    - Describe your removal technique
    - How do you manage break-through bleeding?
- What are the non-contraceptive benefits of the Nexplanon?
- How does Nexplanon differ from Implanon?

Intrauterine Device (IUD)
- How does the IUD work?
- How do you select patient for an IUD?
- What if the IUD string is not visible?
- What is your management if an IUD user becomes pregnant?
    First trimester
    Second trimester
- What are the risks to the. . .
    Pregnancy
    Fetus
- When should an IUD be removed?
- What are complications of IUD?
- Describe the different IUDs available.
- What are the non-contraceptive benefits of an IUD?
- A patient with an IUD needs a LEEP. How do you manage?
- A patient with an IUD needs an endometrial biopsy. How do you manage?
- Are IUDs recommended in women with a history of an ectopic?

Oral Contraceptive Pills (OCPs)
- Which pill formulation is best for treatment for acne?
- Which pill formulation is best for treatment for PMDD?
- Which formulations will induce amenorrhea?
- What are relative and absolute contraindications?
- Which are the best for prevention or reduction of physiologic ovarian cysts?
- What are the non-contraceptive benefits of OCPs?
- Discuss the role of OCPs in the following medical conditions:
    migraine headache
    systemic lupus
    h/o thromboembolism
    smoker

Polycystic Ovarian Syndrome (PCOS)
- Define PCOS per Rotterdam criteria.
- What is the patient presentation?
- What is the laboratory work up?
- What is the source of estrogen in a patient with PCOS?
- How to treat PCOS in a patient who does not desire pregnancy?
- How to treat PCOS in a patient who does desire pregnancy?
- What is metabolic syndrome?
- Discuss hirsutism vs virilization.
- What are the androgens in which organ are they produced?
- What meds have androgenic activity?
- What is the role of 5-alpha reductase?
- How is testosterone carried in the circulation?

- How does this change in response to increased androgens?
    - Increased estrogens?
- What are the non-pharmacologic and pharmacologic treatment options for hirsutism?
- How does late-onset congenital adrenal hyperplasia (CAH) differ from at birth?
- How is CAH diagnosed?
- What is the treatment for CAH?

Abnormal Uterine Bleeding (AUB)
- Discuss the norms for each of the following regarding the menstrual cycle:
    - Frequency
    - Duration
    - Flow
- Define
    - Heavy menstrual bleeding (HMB)
    - Intermenstrual bleeding (IMB)
- Define each of the PALM-COEIN Classification System
    - Structural Causes
        - P
        - A
        - L
        - M
    - Nonstructural Causes
        - C
        - O
        - E
        - I
        - N
- What is differential diagnosis per age group?
    - Adolescence
    - Reproductive
    - Menopausal
- How would you work up each age group? Discuss how each of the following differ between age groups:
    - Medical History
    - Physical Exam
    - Labs
    - Imaging
    - Sampling
- When is imaging indicated?
- What is your threshold for sampling for sonographic endometrial stripe thickness in pre- vs. post-menopause?
- What treatment options are available for each diagnosis above?
- What is your treatment for acute HMB?
- Why are oral contraceptives effective for AUB?

- Are IUDs useful for the treatment of AUB?
- What invasive/surgical treatments are available for AUB? How do you select one for your patient?

IV. Other

Drugs
- brand and generic name, components (especially for OCPs and HRT), mechanism of action, indications/contraindications, administration (dose, duration), side effects, antidote

Labs
- units, indications, interpretation, effect of timing of lab draw on results

TABLE 8.2 "Hot Topics"

1. Obstetrics

Infections: For each infection, discuss the following:
   What is the causative organism?
   Are there vectors?
   How do you detect the infection?
   What is the risk of transmission to the fetus and does that vary per trimester?
   What are the fetal and maternal manifestations?
   How do you treat the fetus and the mom?
   Is a vaccine available and when can you give it?
   Does the infection affect the timing and route of delivery?
   What is the treatment?
   How do you recognize and treat sepsis?
      TORCH Infections
          Toxoplasmosis
          Rubella
          Cytomegalovirus
          Herpes Simplex Virus
   Varicella
   Group B Beta Streptococcus
   Group A Streptococcus
   Syphilis
   Hepatitis B & C
   Fifth's disease
   HIV
   UTI, Pyelonephritis, Asymptomatic bacteria
   Cholecystitis
   Appendicitis
   Chorioamnionits
   Endometritis

Vaginal birth after cesarean section (VBAC): TOLAC candidates, contraindicated, counseling risks/benefits, labor management, recognition/management of uterine rupture.

Isoimmunization, nonimmune hydrops – recognition, management, Rhogam, MCA dopplers

Post dates: definition, management (when and how to induce)

Prolonged rupture of membranes – when to induce

Preterm rupture of membranes – affect of gestational age on management, organisms, antibiotics, diagnosis of chorioamnionits

Forceps vs. vacuum: outlet vs. low vs. mid, indications for each, how long to pull, types of fetal trauma

Induction of labor: cervical ripening, pitocin protocols, IUPCs

Preterm labor: risk factors, causes, management (steroids, tocolytics, fibronectin), management in subsequent pregnancy (17OH Progesterone, cervical length, fibronectin)

Intrauterine growth retardation: symmetric vs. asymmetric, causes

Multifetal pregnancy: chorion/amnion status (diagnosis, clinical significance), twin-to-twin transfusion (diagnosis, management), antepartum management, presentation and delivery options

Bleeding in pregnancy: first-trimester vs. second-trimester vs. third-trimester

    Placenta abruption – risk factors, diagnosis, antepartum/intrapartum management (DIC, blood replacement

    Placenta previa/accreta – risk factors, diagnosis, antepartum management, intraoperative management, complications/sequale

Thromboembolic Disorders – Risk factors, especially inheritable, work-up, prophylaxis, diagnosis and management (including heparin, low molecular weight heparin, coumadin) of DVT and pulmonary embolus

FHR Management: recognition on FHR monitor strips: Category I, II, III, differential diagnosis of causes, management

Antepartum testing: non-stress test, contraction stress test, biophysical profile

Preconception counseling: counseling options – cell-free DNA, Nuchal translucency, CVS, amniocentesis, ultrasound, soft markers, maternal serum screening, integrative, sequential

Episiotomy: routine vs indicated, type – midline vs. mediolateral, complications -3rd, 4th repair

Cesarean delivery: maternal request – counseling; multiple repeats – antepartum management, counseling, intraoperative management including Cesarean hysterectomy

Cancer in pregnancy: breast cancer, cervical cancer, ovarian cancer; presentation, work up, management per trimester, maternal issues, fetal issues

II. Gynecology

Hysteroscopy: counseling, technique, diagnostic vs. operative (distending media, management of I/O discrepancy)

Leiomyomata: symptoms, evaluation, treatment (medical vs hysteroscopic vs embolization) vs surgery – selection of route of hysterectomy, pre/intra-operative measures to decrease bleeding

Pelvic inflammatory disease – causative organisms, presentation, outpatient vs inpatient management, antibiotics, surgical management

Sterilization – counseling, types (hysteroscopic occlusion, postpartum, laparoscopic

Laparoscopic tubal ligation: failure, technique, issues for reversal, anesthesia risks

Oncology—especially cervical, ovarian, uterine: presentation, work up, when to refer, when to stage

Endometrial hyperplasia: significance of atypia, office endometrial sampling vs. D&C, hormonal vs. surgical treatment, uterine cancer

Abnormal cervical cytology: role of HPV, Gardasil, influence of age on management, ASCUS, AGUS, colposcopy technique and interpretation, LEEP vs CKC, management of involved margins

Ectopic pregnancy: work up, diagnosis (ultrasound, HCGs), medical management (candidates, methotrexate- mechanism of action, dosing, surveillance, complications), surgical management (laparoscopy vs laparotomy, salpingectomy vs salpingostomy)

Laparoscopy: technique, safety, types of injury (GI, vascular, ureter)

Blood replacement therapy: indications, PRBCs, FFP, cryoprecipitate

Thromboembolic Disorders: risk factors, especially inheritable, work-up, prophylaxis, diagnosis and management (including heparin, how molecular weight heparin, coumadin) of DVT and pulmonary embolus

Bladder Injuries – prevention, recognition – intraoperative vs postoperative, management – intraoperative and postoperative, duration of drainage

Gastrointestinal injuries- prevention, recognition, management of bowel injury (intra-op, post-operative: SBO vs ileus – work up, radiologic findings, management)

Post op wound complications – recognition (seroma, cellulites, dehiscence, evisceration, necrotizing fasciitis), management

Postop fever: differential diagnosis, work-up, management

Endometriosis: pathophysiology, presentation, work up, medical management (OCPs, progesterone, GnRH agonists), surgical management (intraoperative findings, approach), postoperative management

Chronic pelvic pain: differential diagnosis, work up, treatment

Perioperative coexisting medical problems (respiratory, cardiac, diabetes, electrolyte disturbances, anticoagulation) – screening, work up, when to get preoperative clearance, when to postpone surgery, management of medications (coumadin, oral hypoglycemics, insulin, anti-hypertensives), postoperative complications, life-threatening management

Procidentia: work-up and surgical approach, prevention

Stress urinary incontinence: work-up (standing stress test, Q-tip test), differentiate from urge incontinence, management (surgical vs. conservative), surgical technique, management of intra/post operative complications

III. Office Practice

Abnormal lactation: presentation, work-up (labs, MRI, x-ray), treatment, management in pregnancy

Primary/Secondary Amenorrhea: presentation, work-up (including congenital abnormalities: Mayer Rokitansky Kuster-Hauser Syndrome, testicular feminization, Turner's), causes, treatment

Precocious and delayed puberty: normal puberty, definitions, causes, work up, treatment

Breast disease:
   breast lump – physical exam, work up, breast cyst aspiration (technique, what to do depending upon type of aspirate – bloody, golden, green, dry aspirate) management, when to refer

   breast discharge – physical exam, work up and management depending upon type of discharge: milky, bloody, clear, green, golden

Chronic pelvic pain: differential diagnosis, work up

Basic infertility: up to and including clomid

Premenstrual dysphoric disorder (PMDD), PMS, depression: diagnosis, treatment (medications, alternatives)

Ambiguous genitalia (congenital adrenal hyperplasia): normal sexual development, presentation, work up, causes, definitions

Primary Care: Screening, diagnosis, initial management, criteria for referral

   HTN – diagnosis, definition, anti-hypertensive medications

   Diabetes – screening, diagnosis, medications (oral vs insulin)

   Thyroid disease – (Hyper- and Hypo-) presentation, work-up (labs), treatment (thyroid replacement, PTU)

   Dyslipidemia – screening (labs), treatment (medications, alternatives)

   Gastrointestinal disease – chronic constipation, irritable bowel syndrome, diarrhea, dyspepsia, PUD

   Respiratory tract disease: asthma, community acquired pneumonia, tuberculosis

Menopause: HRT (risks vs. benefits; defense of your drug preference; knowledge of specific hormone content), WHI study

Osteoporosis: risk factors, bone density (interpretation, Z vs. T score), treatment

Endometriosis –pathogenesis, presentation, work up, medical management (OCPs, progesterone, GnRH agonists)

Obesity: BMI, counseling, treatment (medications and alternatives)

Smoking cessation: counseling, treatment

Substance abuse: recognition, counseling, work-up

Sexual dysfunction: types, counseling, treatment

Vulvar disease: differential diagnosis chancre, vulvar dystrophy, skin cancer (malignant melanoma)

Urinary incontinence: overactive bladder – work-up, treatment (medical vs bladder training), stress urinary incontinence – Kegels

Prolapse: pessaries

Sexual assault: state requirements, collection or evidence, STD testing and treatment, emergency contraception, counseling

Intimate partner violence: recognition, counseling (escape plan), state requirements

Another means by which to study various topics is through reviewing gross and microscopic pathology. Historically, they have been an integral part of our training since medical school. They even were formerly a component of the oral board exam, but they were deleted in the mid-1990s.

Until 1997, the ABOG Bulletin stated that interpretation of "gross and microscopic pathology" was fair game. However, subsequent Bulletins eliminated this specific verbiage and replaced it with "interpretation of sonograms, operating videos and videographics of various conditions".

For the sake of being thorough, I have included a list of topics and their accompanying microscopic slides (Table 8.3), should you want to complete an exhaustive review. Time is precious; I would not prioritize the study of pathology. In fact, I dare say that I wouldn't study them at all.

TABLE 8.3 Pathology Microscopic Slides

Fallopian Tube
  Salpingitis
  Salpingitis isthmica
  Ectopic pregnancy
Vagina
  Adenosis
  Clear cell adenocarcinoma
Vulva
  VIN III
  Vulvar dystrophy; lichen sclerosus and squamous hyperplasia
  Papillary hidradenoma
  Squamous cell carcinoma
  Extra-mammary Paget's disease
  Condylomata
Cervix
  Sqaumous cell carcinoma
  HGSIL
  Condylomata
Uterus
  Leiomyomata
  Adenomyosis
  Proliferative endometrium
  Complex adenomatous hyperplasia vs. atypia
  Adenocarcinoma
  Hydatidiform mole
Ovary
  Mucinous cystadenoma or cystadenocarcinoma
  Serous cystadenoma or cystadenocarcinoma
  Brenner's tumor
  Dysgerminoma
  Granulosa cell
  Mature cystic tertoma
  Endometriosis

In conclusion, have a written study plan. Prioritize it based on exam probability, your personal strengths and weaknesses and topics generated by your case list. Reevaluate your plan as needed and draft an updated plan accordingly. Confine your study to a clinically oriented review. Acknowledge that it is impossible to study everything on your list. Finally, don't forget to take breaks to avoid burnout.

Mock Oral Exams

You can study all you want, but if you can't articulate what you know, you simply will not pass this test. Rarely have I met an individual who can pull this off without practice. Most of you will strategically postpone the inevitable until the last minute. Why would you spend a year collecting cases, study for months, and then scrimp with mock oral exams, the most important study tool of all?

I have mentored candidates preparing for their oral board exam for nearly twenty five years. I feel it takes only three mock oral exams for most to become comfortable with this mode of examination. Just like any new skill, the learning curve is exponential.

Besides, let's give credit where credit is due. Admit it—you simply could not have made it this far if you were not pretty clever. Come on, you made it through MCATs, medical school, USMLEs, residency, CREOG in-service training exams and the written boards. You are one smart dude. However, what was the most common test format for all of these? Yup, that's right, the written exam. So trust me on this one. You must experience some mock oral exams. You will be ever so glad you did. Now let me show you how.

First, let's start with the one examiner to whom you have ready access… namely YOU! Don't underestimate yourself at all. As a matter of fact, you will be the toughest guy to get past. I conduct oral exam workshops; and right away, we put you in the examiner's seat. Everyone comments about how they totally underestimated how helpful another candidate can be.

You are helpful in two ways. First, look at your or another candidate's case list. What would you ask if you were the examiner? At the workshop, the most popular session is when we allow you to present your nightmare case. Everyone gets to fire any possible question they foresee. We have determined it takes just six to eight minutes to flush out all questions. Hands down unanimous, the questions predicted in this session were indeed asked on the actual exam.

Secondly, quiz yourself out loud. Refer back to those Know Cold topics, such as vaginal breech delivery, that we just discussed earlier in this chapter. Write out the management on an index card and by rote, memorize the answer. You can post these on your bathroom mirror or take them with you in the car on your commute or use them when you exercise.

Now practice out loud alone. You must get familiar with answering out loud, rather than silently. Unfortunately, you don't sound nearly as eloquent out loud as you do in your head. Now practice in front of the mirror. YIKES! Would you trust that guy delivering your vaginal breech? Practice until the answer is a resounding yes.

OK, now involve your loved ones. You really need their support during this trying time. They will so much more buy into the whole gig if you enlist their aid. Practice your rote answer to your spouse. They don't need to know a darn thing about a vaginal breech delivery. However, it is ever so helpful to now use another person as a sounding board. Give them your index cards, so they can follow along. They will readily pick up and let you know if you left anything out. Let's stay in your comfort zone; now enlist your partner's help. At this point, you don't have to make a big deal out it. Just ask them to listen to your answer as you are closing on an abdominal case or in the doctor's lounge in between cases.

Now it's time to get some mock oral exams on defending your case list. No, this is not a review; nor is it a way to troubleshoot anticipated topics, but it is an actual mock oral exam. That means you need to use the case list that you submitted to ABOG; yes, the one that lacks all your crib notes. I strongly advocate tapping into some local and regional colleagues. There is a tendency to procrastinate, as you will probably feel you are not ready. Yet, you will probably never be ready, if you go by your standards. Besides, you don't want to be embarrassed by acknowledging you don't know everything. Guess what? Your colleagues already know you don't know everything, because they don't either! Remember, you are at your knowledge peak. You will probably never know so much about so much again! So give yourself a break and just dive on in. I guarantee that not one single colleague will decline your request to give you a mock oral exam. It is such an honor to help another colleague.

So what are some examples of local and regional colleagues? Local colleagues are those right there in your community where you practice. This would include partners in your group, those that you share call with, or other generalists in your town.

Regional colleagues are typically those subspecialists to whom you refer your patients. This is a great opportunity to get to know them, since most of the time you're communicating by phone. A bonus is to remember that your examiner will most likely be a subspecialist, so it is nice to get their perspective, especially if you are a generalist. So have your referring MFM quiz you on your obstetrics case list, your gyn oncologist or urogynecologist on your gynecology list and your REI on your office case list.

Definitely your local and regional colleagues are plentiful, readily available and at the right price. However, you get what you pay for. If they do not routinely give mock oral exams, then their only experience will most likely be their own oral board exam. An n = 1 in any study is of very limited value. So give them the following guidelines and instructions, so they can be the most helpful.

1. Ideally review my case list ahead of time and pick out the top ten cases.
2. Let's start with those top ten cases – you can tell me later why those were of interest to you.
3. Do you mind if I record this? Here let me quickly set up my cell phone. Don't worry, I've got it aimed on me, but my wife/husband/partner tells me I have this crazy nervous tic. I want to see for myself. Besides, even though I know you, I still get nervous and I can't remember the questions and responses for later review.
4. I brought a stop watch. Let's go for ten minutes straight, then later twenty, then ultimately for thirty minutes like on the test.
5. I really appreciate your help, but do not interrupt to give me feedback. We'll do that after our designated time.
6. You're going to love this, but don't be nice to me. It doesn't help at all. Put on your best poker face. No feedback, no encouragement, no smiling, no nodding of the head, no nothing.
7. Please write down my answers. That will help to keep us both on track with the line of questioning, plus it simulates the exam. I can also refer to your notes when I review the recording.

Another pool of mock oral examiners is academicians – both past and present. Call the residency director of the closest residency. I'm sure either he and/or his faculty would be happy to help you out. Why not make a trip back to where you did your residency and meet with your residency director or some of your favorite faculty? Better yet, choose that one faculty that was always so tough on you. Yeah, the malignant one … he's perfect. Don't assume that they have experience in mock oral exams. Remember, they were preparing you for the written boards. You may need to give them the above guidelines too.

Another source of mock orals is the internet via webinar. They are of some, albeit limited, value. Obviously, there is no face-to-face contact, so it in no way comes close to simulating the anxiety in looking the examiner directly in the eye. It is helpful in that you get to practice with someone who doesn't know you, so they have no reason to cut you any slack. Additionally, you get to compare yourself to others and seek to emulate those who performed well.

The tutorial and workshops are another good source. Like the webinars, they share similar pros/cons. The best feature is the one-on-one exposure. These are helpful even if it's another colleague, as afterwards you can commiserate and hopefully even connect with some newfound study buddies. I'm not a fan of group public mock orals as they are on the verge of degrading. They bring back flashbacks of M&M and other adversarial torture. Most find it really hard to think when a bunch of eyes are staring back at you. Besides, this doesn't accurately reflect the exam setting, since you will, thankfully, only have two examiners and not a room full.

Finally, I recommend you take at least one mock oral exam with a professional. This is someone who is remunerated for providing this service, so typically a faculty from a review or tutorial course. Do not assume that just because they are being paid they are qualified. Verify their credentials, experience, track record and especially, that they are a clinician. A past board examiner is the ultimate, unless of course, he is no longer practicing medicine.

After you have taken a few mock oral exams, you will appreciate the tricks your mind will play. The biggest and final obstacle to overcome is YOU. If you truly believe you will pass this exam, then you will. Believe in yourself!

Mind your mind. Envision the whole process, starting with your arrival in Dallas. Put your suit on, look at yourself and emblazon the image in your mind. Now put yourself in the exam room. Envision the examiners and you answering their questions thoughtfully, confidently and quickly. Set yourself up for success. Make it so!

In conclusion, you cannot attempt this exam unprepared. You have to be book smart, but you must also be able to persuasively articulate this knowledge. I suppose any ole' mock oral exam is better than no mock oral exam. However, you will excel quicker if you give your mock oral examiners guidelines on how to best help you. Practice doesn't make perfect. Rather, *perfect practice* makes perfect. Practice for the real thing. Anything less is second best.

Chapter 9

Image Enhancement

You can't judge a book by its cover—or can you? Image enhancement is a facet of testmanship that is traditionally ignored. It entails the strategy of optimizing not what you say, but how you say it. In other words, it is how to influence positively, or manipulate, the examiner's first impression.

Stereotypically, physicians ignore society's emphasis on the physical impression, whereas in other professions (such as business or law), one's image can make or break a deal or case. A well-known study concluded that the first impression is based predominantly (55%) on appearance. Second, the quality of one's voice, such as tone, pitch and speech pattern, has a 38% influence. A mere 7% is based on what you say. Furthermore, the first impression is made within only five seconds.

Some of you may argue that you don't have to, that you don't want to, and ultimately that you refuse to play the game. But given all the effort that has gone into preparing for this exam, can you really afford not to? Why not approach this issue as stacking the deck? Not bucking the system, but beating the system. Besides, if you don't like it, change it when you're the examiner. Remember, "You can't change the system if you're not in the system."

Testmanship is the art of knowing not only what is on the exam, but who the examiner is.

An examiner's academic profile influences the type of questions that he or she asks. Similarly, understanding the examiner's physical image will give you yet another insight into his or her makeup. The more you know about the examiners, the better armed you are to battle with them.

Most examiners are leaders in their field. This status usually dictates frequent public and peer exposure and henceforth, conformity to a stereotypic dress code. Furthermore, the majority are male and middle-aged; however, increasingly, more are women. Stereotypically, they dress conservatively. Typical attire for a male examiner is khaki pants, a navy sport coat and a button-down shirt with a bow-tie or a paisley or striped tie. A female examiner will be similarly conservatively attired in a pant or skirt suit.

I want to reiterate the importance of the first impression made by your case list. Remember, the examiner has already reviewed your case list before he meets you. He has a mental image of you based solely on your case list. When the examiner actually meets you, he or she will quickly see if the impression matches. This is the time - and you only have five seconds —to either solidify a positive impression or persuade the examiner to reconsider if he or she has misjudged you.

Let's now walk through the components involved in the first five critical seconds with the examiner. The most influential is appearance. The two most important components of appearance are tailoring and color. Tailoring should capitalize on your positive physical features and downplay the negative. For example, if you are overweight, choose clothes that make you look more lean. Simply lengthening the tie distracts from a protuberant abdomen. I recommend that men wear a suit and tie. A sport coat, although collegiate, is not as professional as a two-piece suit.

For women, the theme is conservative, yet feminine and fashionable, clothes. Appropriate attire is either a dress or a two-piece suit (pant or skirt). A skirt or slacks and blouse without a jacket is too plain and not as professional.

Color can make an impact, either negative or positive. An inexpensive investment that lasts a lifetime is to have your colors professionally analyzed. Many companies offer a trained image consultant who, with the help of computer analysis, can determine your most complimentary colors. Extensive research is available to determine what impact certain colors will make.

Safe colors for your suit are blue, black or brown. Grey, which is a common color, is rarely flattering for most, unless you have black or grey hair. A suit that matches your hair color makes the whole package flow. A blouse or shirt that matches your skin tone is the most flattering. If you really want to wow them, match your eye color and that will pull them right in for some direct eye contact. Although it may seem trite, candidates who use the right colors will be at a clear advantage.

The basics—hose, socks, shoes and belt—should complement, not compete with, your outfit. For men, the socks should match the pant color. For women, the hose should do the same; if the outfit is dark, wear black, blue or gray hose. Pastel or bold colors are best complemented by neutral hose. The color of the shoes and belt should match and tastefully blend with the outfit's colors.

Accessories are the icing on the cake. If worn tastefully, they can complement an outfit and add sophistication and flare. On the other hand, gaudy, expensive jewelry or ill-matched accessories are distracting. The only acceptable piercings are in the ears. Sorry guys, you don't get to wear any earrings; and ladies, limit yours to no more than two per ear. Jewelry should be understated yet sophisticated. Ties and scarves are a wonderful asset to express individuality, as well as to capitalize on your best colors and good taste.

Hairstyle has a great effect on your appearance. For men, the length of hair is particularly important. You are trying to uphold the image of a clean-cut, well-groomed, board-certified obstetrician and gynecologist. This does not mean that you cannot have a beard or mustache, but if you do, it must be trimmed and orderly. For women, long hair pulled back by a barrette or in a high pony tail may be seen as girlish and therefore, unprofessional.

My final comments about appearance are trivial, but help you to score points for style and attention to detail, such as using the term "leiomyomata" instead of fibroids. Fingernails should be clean and well manicured. If you chose to wear polish, it should be neutral and non-assuming. Since you are a surgeon, your hands reflect your craft and are an indirect measure of how meticulous you are in the operating room.

Look carefully at your shoes. Make sure they are polished and not scuffed. Treat yourself to a professional shoe shine in the airport when you are en route to your exam. Likewise, your belt buckle should be polished without areas of worn leather. Women should wear low heels—not high heels and not flats.

Don't underestimate the appearance of even your case list. At a minimum, staple the pages, so you don't accidentally trip and scatter it all over the floor. Better yet, organize it into a three-ringed binder and you can even put each page in a sleeve. The classiest touch of all is to have your copy professionally bound.

Appearance accounts for the majority of the first impression. The next factor, before you have even spoken one word, is the handshake. Because this is admittedly a stressful situation, you may well have cold and clammy hands. If they are like ice cubes, stuff them into your pockets beforehand. Your handshake should be firm but not bone-breaking. Women also should avoid a weak or limp-wristed handshake. You should look the examiner squarely in the eyes to project confidence, and smile, albeit nervously.

The second most influential component of the first impression is voice quality. Because a first impression is made in only five seconds, the introduction is critical. Be aware of how anxiety and nervousness affect your speech. Practice the introduction until it is calm and projects confidence.

Consider standing out from the vast majority who will reflexively respond, "Nice to meet you" upon being introduced to the examiner. Instead, how about "It's an honor or privilege to meet you"? A personal touch would be to add the examiner's name.

In conclusion, you cannot afford to underestimate the power of the first impression. Your case list has already evoked an initial mental image. The first five seconds of meeting you, however, leave a lasting impression. Attention to your image is merely another facet of testmanship. Strategizing how to enhance your image is as important as strategizing how to convey your knowledge. It is capitalizing on the age-old saying, "It's not what you say, but how you say it." Remember, you never get a second chance to make a great first impression.

Chapter 10
The Oral Exam

Until 2000, all of the exams were conducted over the course of one week at the Westin Hotel in Chicago, and typically held in early November. Since 2000, the exams have been administered in Dallas and are spread out over three months. The candidates are divided into three groups and each group is examined over one week in each of three months: November, December and January. The reason for this change is not clear. It certainly makes exam security a lot tougher, and major holidays —Thanksgiving, Christmas/Hanukkah and New Years—are definitely ruined. Perhaps the board intends to use the same pool of examiners for all three months to promote standardization and consistency of exam conduct and thus, afford truer assessment of pass/fail.

In the past, it was rumored that a minimum percentage of candidates were designated for failure. This change refutes that rumor because the results of the exams are announced within one week. Obviously the November results cannot be delayed until the January exams. Whatever the reasons for the change, it does not change your timeline for preparation. Once you know the date of your exam, back-plot the timeline for studying as recommended in Table 1 of Chapter 4, "Getting Started". Given that the December and January dates coincide with the holidays, don't dillydally in making your airline reservations to Dallas.

The Day Before

I strongly recommend you read Chapter 12, "A Candidate's Journey", both before and after you read the rest of this chapter to capture the emotions and stress experienced going into the exam. No matter how well you have prepared, you will be nervous ... *very* nervous. You must acknowledge your anxiety and understand how this anxiety affects your performance, to truly be able to take the bull by the horns. To pretend that this is just another day at the office, or that you're having a casual collegial discussion is foolhardy, naïve and very risky.

I recommend that you arrive in Dallas at least one or preferably, two days before your exam. While you are traveling, make sure to carry one copy of your case list and your suit with you, just in case the airline loses your luggage. Likewise, tuck a copy of your case list in your luggage, in case you lose or damage the copy that you are hand-carrying. You need a buffer to account for unexpected travel delays. This is especially true if your exam is in December or January, given the unpredictability of winter weather. Most of you will travel great distances and change time zones. You need time to recover and adapt.

Dallas is the home of ABOG and the oral exams are conducted at the ABOG Test Center. The ABOG Diplomate reports that the test center has rooms designed specifically to accommodate the format of the oral exam. These accommodations include high-resolution computer screens with the capability of projecting images and Case of the Day. The screens are intended to "improve the image of the clinical condition under discussion". In the past, a projector for 35-mm slides was set up in the hotel room and images were projected onto the blank wall.

The ABOG Diplomate also reports that candidates will be housed in hotels within a six- to eight-block radius of the test center. The majority of the candidates stay at the Melrose Hotel, simply because ABOG has contracted with them. However, you don't have to stay there at all. Admittedly, it's a bit nerve wracking to see ashen white-faced candidates stumble into the hotel lobby right after the test.

Regardless of your housing options, I recommend you stay within a ten minute walking distance of the Melrose, because you are required to report there the day of your exam. It is critical to be within a quick jaunt in case you forget your case list, or the weather or traffic bogs you down.

Regardless of where you stay, the night before should be spent trying to relax. Do not attempt last-minute cramming. If you feel compelled to do so, skim over your case list. However, this is not the time for a night on

Chapter 10 • The Oral Exam

the town. Try to get a good night's sleep. If you need a sleeping pill, make sure you have tried it before to avoid a hangover for a morning exam. Set your unaltered case list and admission pass somewhere where you will all but trip over them the next morning. Remember, the case list you bring with you to the exam must be IDENTICAL to the one submitted in August. It cannot include any notes, alterations, edits, etc.

The Morning of

On the day of the exam, make sure you eat. Although you are nervous, hypoglycemia will prevent you from performing at your peak. Although it seems obvious, don't eat in your suit, in case an unexpected clumsy waiter drops your food and drink into your lap. After you've eaten, take time to primp. If you look good, you feel good. Dress conservatively and professionally. Use an anxiolytic if necessary, but make sure you have previously tested its side effects. If you have a good-luck charm, by all means tuck it in your pocket.

Don't forget your case list, a picture I.D. and your admission pass. You may not bring cellular phones, computers, reference materials or briefcases to the registration, orientation or testing center. If you are not in walking distance, allow ample time for potential traffic delays.

On the day of your exam, report to the Melrose Hotel at your designated time. Do not be late, as they will lock the doors promptly, in spite of your pounding to let you in. Each day there are two sessions, one in the morning and one in the afternoon. Each session is preceded by a buffet breakfast or lunch.

Typically, there are 30 to 50 candidates per session. Following the meal, the ABOG Executive Director greets and welcomes you. He gives a friendly, uplifting, pep talk to reassure you that you are all smart and this is the most unimportant exam you will take.

You are then called up to receive your specific exam room number. You are requested to turn off and check in any cell phones, computers, recorders and any other electronic devices. Thereafter, the presence of the above devices will be cause for immediate dismissal from the exam. You are allowed to bring a breast pump and a pacemaker. Finally, you sign a declaration of "unrestricted privileges" and receive your photo ID badge. All of the candidates are then shuttled the short distance from the Melrose Hotel to the ABOG testing center—about a 10-15 minute ride.

Upon reaching the ABOG testing center, you are greeted by other cordial and empathetic ABOG dignitaries. The first dignitary gives you an overview of the exam process by showing a 5 minute vignette of the conduct of the exam. The next speaker, usually the Director of Evaluation, tries to break the ice. He spends about 45 minutes with a humorous PowerPoint presentation, further expounding on what to, and what not to, expect. This includes dispelling myths, misperceptions, pass/fail statistics and when to expect your results.

You then get to take a break and go to the bathroom. You definitely want to complete this necessity, as this is your last chance until after the test. Although you can theoretically go to the bathroom during the test, the clock does not stop. You will waste precious time and you will want every single second to prove yourself. You are then instructed to go upstairs to the testing area.

Once there, you will report to your designated exam room. You remain in the same room while each pair of examiners rotates. The rooms are pleasant, well lighted and most have a window. You will sit on a rolling chair on the window side of the desk, facing toward the door. On one side of the desk is a flat-screen monitor, as well as a pad of paper and a pen. The corner of the screen has a clock with the real time. The examiners sit across from you at a tilt podium desk, which contains their keyboard and papers. To your right, there is a pitcher of water and a box of tissue.

The first pair of examiners will enter and introduce themselves. You will then be shown a list of your six examiners, to see if you have any conflicts. Just because you recognize some reputable and distinguished names, or even interviewed with them, does not indicate a true conflict. However, if you perceive a conflict, you should let them know so they can replace that examiner. The test begins promptly at the sound of the computer chime.

Exam Content

The exam is divided into three sections: obstetrics, gynecology, and office practice.

Within each section, there are two categories: the case list and case of the day.

Half of your exam is spent defending your case list, which reflects your mode of practice. The examiner can either refer to specific patients on your case list or use it as a springboard for other topics.

The other category is "structured cases" or "case of the day". The "case of the day" is my term for the written narrative of a hypothetical patient management scenario. Each case of the day requires a standardized response. Although examiners may vary in their approach to each question, this format lends some objectivity to an otherwise predominantly subjective test. On any one day, all candidates will have the same structured cases.

Exam Format

The exam is three hours, divided into three 60 minute blocks - one for each of the three sections: obstetrics, gynecology, and office practice. The 60-minute sessions can occur in any sequence. Half of each of the 60-minute sessions is devoted to your case list and the other half to the case of the day. Effective in 2008, everyone started with, and completed, all of the case of the day discussions before switching to the case list.

There are three pairs of examiners - one pair for each section. Typically, you are questioned by only one examiner at a time. The other observes and documents the conduct of the exam. The exam is also monitored by closed circuit television with sound, but not recorded. One examiner will question you about the case of the day and the other will question you about the case list. At the completion of each 60-minute segment, a chime sounds and the pair of examiners finish, stand up, wish you well and leave. Within one minute, the next pair of examiners will enter.

Although you are sitting for your general boards, traditionally the examiners are subspecialists. Usually the examiner is a specialist in maternal-fetal medicine for the obstetrics section, a reproductive endocrinologist for office practice, and an oncologist or less likely, a FPM for the gynecologic section. Some of the examiners are generalists who can examine any of the three sections.

At any time during the exam, you are allowed to get up and go to the bathroom. To do this is not to your advantage, as the clock does not stop. You also may make notes on the scratch pad which is provided for you. Since you will be referring constantly to your case list, I recommend you organize it into a 3-ring binder with dividers between the 3 sections.

At the end of three hours, the exam is punctually concluded. You make a quick getaway downstairs. You must ride back to the Melrose on the shuttle—no exceptions. Don't cut your escape plans so tight that you miss your flight. Some head straight to the bar at the Melrose.

Evaluation Criteria

The purpose of the exam is to assess your ability to manage patients. The basis for patient management scenarios is derived from your case list, the case of the day and hypothetical patients. The *Bulletin* cites the following generic criteria for evaluation:

1. Develop a diagnosis, including the appropriate clinical, laboratory and diagnostic procedures
2. Select and apply proper treatment, under elective and emergency conditions
3. Prevent, recognize and manage complications
4. Plan and direct follow-up and continuing care

The examination is designed to evaluate your qualifications as a specialist or consultant to non- obstetrician-gynecologist colleagues. The goal of the test is also to evaluate your behavior in independent practice. The emphasis is on patient management knowledge and skills.

The grading system is another coveted secret. The best benchmark or standard to emulate is the ACOG standards. As long as your management is consistent with the ACOG guidelines in the Compendium, you will meet the passing criteria.

Examiner Alerts

Your examiners are supposed to conduct the exam in a fair and unprejudiced fashion. Some do better than others in heeding this directive. Nonetheless, they are all on a mission to "bring the cream to the top". Contrary to popular belief, their goal is to *pass* you. Unlike the written exam, the oral format strips control of the conduct of the exam from you and gives it to the examiner. An out-of-control rookie will undoubtedly crash and burn if not experienced and prepared.

The examiners write continuously. Do not misinterpret this as a poor performance. They are legally required to document the conduct of the exam in case of a dispute.

Examiners change topics abruptly once you have satisfactorily answered their question. They will even curtly interrupt you in the middle of a sentence to move on to the next topic. Don't misinterpret this as rudeness. Quite the contrary, they are doing you a favor to move as quickly as possible. They have only thirty short minutes for each section. The more questions you answer right, the more you will dilute the wrong ones, and obviously enhance your chances for passing.

Chapter 10 • The Oral Exam

Examiners will give you no feedback whatsoever. They will try to conceal facial, postural or verbal gestures and to mask their approval or disapproval. In spite of this stiff environment, they usually are cordial and empathetic—except one.

Consistently there seems to be a "bad guy" in one of the three sections. ABOG formally denies the "good cop, bad cop" innuendos in the introductory slide show. I truly believe there is no designated hit man. However, think back to your residency. Name six faculty members. Bet'cha at least one is not known for his ooey-gooey sweet nature. It took you awhile to just accept him for who he was. You learned to look past this facet of his personality. You and his patients learned to be forgiving for his lack of beside personality; after all, he was a great doctor otherwise. Chances are one of your six examiners is going to be malignant, just because that's his nature.

Recently, the exam has not been as adversarial as it was reputed to be in the past. Dr. Norman Gant, the ABOG executive director until 2007, would introduce himself as being from the KGB, or the Kinder and Gentler Board. I believed him. However, you should be prepared for a not-so-friendly foe. It is usually quite obvious who it is. His job is to create a stressful environment to determine your decision-making ability under such conditions.

Because the bad guy cannot witness your performance in an actual life threatening scenario, he can only hope to simulate the same emotional response. Past tactics include openly displaying disagreement or dissatisfaction with your answers and impatience with your lack of quick decisions. He will even add emotion-provoking qualifiers to cloud your decisions—for example, making malpractice innuendoes or describing extreme social circumstances (e.g., emergency cesarean hysterectomy on a nulliparous).

Perhaps current examiners will all have jumped on the kinder, gentler bandwagon. But be prepared in case you don't get a convert. Try to stay focused on the issues and not be sucked into making hasty, careless decisions. Do not panic. Stay calm, cool and collected. The more mock oral exams you experience, the more skilled and desensitized you become with interrogation under hot lights.

Exam Conduct

No doubt, your best preparation for an oral exam is to take mock oral exams. After all, repetition is the mother of learning, and practice makes perfect. Although you can never take too many, I recommend a minimum of three. The learning curve is definitely exponential.

Although you will discover many of the following tips on your own, prior knowledge of them before your first mock oral will save you from having to reinvent the wheel. Seeing is one thing…doing is another. Make sure you get a chance to try these techniques during a few mock oral exams. Don't let your first time be the day of the exam.

Throughout the exam, remember the phrase "when in Rome, do as the Romans do". You are auditioning to join an elite club. *You* want to be one of *them*. Although you may not agree with their selection process, remember you cannot change the system until you are in the system.

The exam is a humbling experience. Most candidates have invested one to two years in preparing for the exam. Your knowledge base of obstetrics and gynecology is at its peak. Although the majority will pass, most will feel like they failed when they leave the room.

You can't help but reflect on what went wrong. Remember, even after you passed a topic, you will often be driven to the point where you don't know. But that's their goal - to make sure you know your limits and are humble enough to call for help. Just because you think you didn't know the answer to many of the questions doesn't mean that you didn't pass the question and ultimately the exam. So, forewarned is forearmed. If you walk out of the exam knowing you passed, that's a bonus.

The most valuable tip is to *answer only the question*. On the surface, this seems obvious. But most of us are used to a written exam where the succinct answer is right there in black and white. You assume your verbal answer is as succinct, but almost always feel the need to qualify your response further. The more you talk, the more you open other related topics. The examiner may have been perfectly satisfied with your answer, but your rambling opened a new topic. Since you brought it up, it's now fair game for discussion.

Listen carefully to the question. If you don't understand it, ask the examiner to repeat or clarify. Don't risk failing a question because of misinterpretation. If the examiner asks a close-ended question—"Did you do this or that?"—give a close-ended response: yes or no. The examiner who wants more information will ask. Try to answer open-ended questions as succinctly as possible. The exception is the topic on which you are well versed. Purposely lead the examiner into what you want to talk about. Undoubtedly, a few mock orals will help tremendously. Bottom line—*answer the question!*

Accept responsibility for the patients on your case list, regardless of who is at fault for dumping on you. The patient is on your case list; therefore, you own her. If it is important to convey injustice, say "When I assumed her care, she was…etc."

Avoid social, racial or religious justification for a mode of practice, unless appropriate. It would be inappropriate to justify your reason for induction of labor because a patient is of a stereotypic demanding religious sect. On the other hand, ordering certain labs because a patient is at risk for a disease because of his or her race or religion would be entirely appropriate.

Similarly, justify a planned breech of standard of care. You may be precluded from following the norm of practice because of limitations within a group practice or hospital facilities. For example, you may not be able to offer methotrexate for nonsurgical management of ectopic pregnancy because you are in the military, deployed overseas and practicing out of a tent! Perhaps you would like to offer laser vaporization of lower genital tract condylomata, but are unable to do so because your rural hospital cannot afford a laser. Nonetheless, if you elect to violate the standard, simply acknowledge your understanding of the standard and support why you cannot adhere to it.

Speaking of standards, the ACOG standard of care is the standard by which you are judged. The ACOG Compendium, which houses the *Practice Bulletins*, *Committee Opinions*, *Technology Assessments, and Safety Checklists* are the best references. Know them! Know what an Ob/Gyn consultant for non-Ob/Gyn practitioners would do—and don't go beyond those boundaries.

Settle the tug of war of "what I do versus what I *should* do" ahead of time. For example, everyone has induced a patient for macrosomia, yet we all know that the ACOG evidence-based guidelines do not support this practice. So hopefully, if you are reading this before August 1, you can avoid this problem in the first place by simply listing it as an elective induction. If you are now in a case list defense mode, acknowledge your understanding of the guidelines and shift the focus on how the patient was counseled.

The examiners are quite clever in pushing you to your limits. Don't say you would do something that normally you would not do. For example, if a complication of your breast cyst aspiration is a pneumothorax and the examiner asks you what the next step is, respond with "insertion of a chest tube". If the examiner wants to know the technique for placing a chest tube and you don't normally place chest tubes (as most of us do not), explain that you would consult your general surgeon and/or emergency department physician.

Once you have acknowledged your limitations, the examiner should back off. Sometimes, however, he or she may resort to below-the-belt tactics and make your consultant unavailable or ask what your consultant would do. This is probably a hint that the examiner expects you to know more and is especially common in discussing intraoperative ureteral injuries. If you truly know what the consultant would do, answer the question. However, emphasize that you are not comfortable performing the procedure independently. If you do not know the answer, hold your ground and say that you will have to wait for the consultant.

Freely admit if you don't know. The examiner would rather hear an acknowledgment of your limitations than a foolhardy guess. If you guess, do so only if you are reasonably sure; otherwise you will discredit yourself. However, you probably know more than what you give yourself credit for. Try to tell them what you do know, so hopefully you can get partial credit.

Don't change your answers. The golden rule for a written exam, "Never change your first answer" also applies to an oral exam. The examiners are skillful at manipulating you so you end up second-guessing your answer. They often put words in your mouth. More cleverly, they will uncharacteristically grant you the opportunity to change your answer. Their encouragement and atypical empathy are just a facade. Their real agenda is to determine whether your decision making is certain and consistent.

Don't be overconfident. Arrogance is frowned upon and viewed in the same negative light as lack of confidence. This exam quickly puts you in your place. Rarely, there may be topics about which you are more knowledgeable than the examiner. Refrain from seizing the opportunity to lecture, teach or argue. This is not the appropriate forum. Given the fact that the examiners are judging you, this is not the time to embarrass or anger them.

Likewise, refrain from saying "the literature" says this or that. The examiner will then ask you to specify exactly what you mean by "the literature"—which journal, the authors and so on. Don't fall into this trap.

On the other hand, you may have indeed modeled a mode of practice after a specific article. It may be appropriate to reveal this, but be prepared to cite the specifics of the article. In addition, this will open the door for questions about how to review the literature critically, such as the power of the study and alpha and beta errors.

Perhaps the most difficult skill to master is to let a question go once you have answered it. Let bygones be bygones. Do not compromise the remaining questions by dwelling on the last one. Remember, you want to answer as many questions as possible, so the right answers will dilute the wrong ones. This is a skill that must be practiced; but once mastered, will definitely be the ace up your sleeve.

Points for Style

The following recommendations will win you points for style. These are subtleties that will raise your favorable impression a notch. They make up the gestalt, the hunch, the gut feeling the examiner has about you.

Listen carefully to the question. If you don't understand it, ask the examiner to repeat or clarify. Don't risk failing a question because of misinterpretation. This is not to be confused with a novice candidate repeating the question with their answer. For example, if I ask you, "What is your differential diagnosis for chronic pelvic pain?", you should reply with the answer. Don't resort to the age-old stall tactic by replying, "What's the differential diagnosis for chronic pelvic pain? The differential diagnosis for chronic pelvic pain is …" You're obviously stalling and thinking out loud. I emphasize again, just answer the question directly.

If you understand the question, but need to ponder the answer, don't be afraid of silence. This is an enormous power play on your part. The ball is in your court. The examiner is powerless to move the exam on until you respond. This is not to be confused as a stall tactic. It is never to your advantage to slow the exam, as you want to answer as many questions as possible. However, being comfortable with silence is a rare trait that portrays a calm, cool and collected candidate. It also assures you don't ramble nonsensically and open up Pandora's Box with unintended new ammunition for the examiner.

Try to maintain eye contact with the examiner. Don't you hate it when someone won't look you in the eye when you're talking to them? What are they trying to hide? What are they afraid of? Don't they have confidence in what they're saying? Obviously, the same questions will be going through the examiner's mind, particularly when he compares you to the other candidates. Again, a few mock orals will fix this easily. I advise those who simply can't make eye contact to at least look directly at the examiner's nose.

Be aware of your posture and body language. Sit poised and natural. Remember, if you are not accustomed to wearing a suit, you should wear it for at least one mock oral exam. Many of us have nervous tics of which we are unaware.

Express your thoughts verbally; after all, this is an oral exam. Do you talk with your hands? Some candidates especially succumb to using their hands to describe a procedure, such as how to deliver a breech vaginally or manage a shoulder dystocia. It's hysterical to watch a novice go through all the gestures and gyrations to demonstrate each maneuver. However, if you can articulate elegantly without supplementing with your hands, you will hands down stand out from the majority.

Be polite and respectful. I know this seems obvious, but I disagree with the advice to treat the examiner casually, like he is your partner or you are having a curbside consult. The oral board exam is anything but a casual affair; this is the biggest test of your career! The examiners are prestigious leaders in our field. I would address him/her respectfully as Doctor. Certainly, if you are comfortable doing so, also add ma'am or sir.

Accept responsibility for the patients on your case list. A common mistake in answering a question is to say "we", such as "we did this, then we did that". Certainly the practice of medicine requires a team approach, especially in the operating room. However, I think you'll agree to say "we did a pap smear" sounds ridiculous. The exam is not a team effort – YOU are the only one sitting in the hot seat. The patient is on *your* case list; therefore, she's *your* patient. Instead of "we", say "I".

Do not say *never* and *always*. These terms imply certainty in the inexact practice of medicine. Likewise, avoid the terms *inadvertently*, *routinely*, *protocol* or *that's how I was trained*. They imply resistance to change or comfort with the modus operandi, which is not the image of an up-to-date, board-certified obstetrician and gynecologist.

Choose your words carefully. Using the word *declines* rather than *refuses* is kinder and implies more neutral and informed counseling. For example, "The patient with a previous low transverse Cesarean section declined a trial of labor". However, you may want to say the patient refused a Cesarean section for a terminal bradycardia fetal heart rate tracing to justify a mid forceps delivery.

The examiners love when you humbly admit you made a mistake; even better is to acknowledge, such as *I learned from this and now I do this*. This is also an effective way to turn the tide in defending an obvious complication on your case list.

The End

A chime will signal the end of each one-hour segment. The examiners will abruptly conclude and stand up to leave. You should also stand up to be respectful and shake their hand. *Smile, look them in the eye* and *thank* them. Have the same firm handshake that you did when they first walked into the room. Remember to make a great lasting impression.

Whatever you do, do not request a repeat exam. The exception would be egregious behavior such as an examiner falling asleep or spending excessive time on one case. According to the ABOG *Bulletin*, if a candidate feels that the exam was not conducted in a fair and unprejudiced manner, he or she may request a repeat exam within one hour of completion of the oral exam.

The examiners are typically experienced with years of examining candidates. It is unlikely that your exam was really conducted unfairly and/or with prejudice. We will discuss how the results are tabulated in the next chapter. However, each pair of examiners independently determines your results. The examiners for one section have no idea as to who the other pair of examiners might be. Use this to your advantage and recover if you bombed one section. Don't compromise the other two sections! Besides, statistically you have about an 85% chance of passing. Those odds are really in your favor.

If you think you did poorly and you will have a better chance the second time around, you have to wait until next year; plus, you have to collect a new case list! The repeat exam is conducted by a different set of examiners who do not know that the candidate appealed.

The oral board exam is the climax of months of preparation. Admittedly, the bulk of your effort is building your knowledge base. The icing on the cake however, is the persuasive articulation of your knowledge.

Few candidates can perform well and comfortably in an oral exam without practice. It's a shame to spend months on studying and not to devote a few hours to mock oral exams. Incorporating the above tips should give you the "razor's edge". With practice, you'll find that the oral exam format is actually easier than the written exam.

Chapter 11
Test Results

Historically, departing remarks were a clue to whether or not you passed the exam. "Have a nice flight" or "Enjoy the holidays" implied that you had passed. There is no more guarantee in these remarks than there is in predicting the sex of a fetus by its heart rate. ABOG dispels this claim in the 45-minute introductory slide show. The specific criteria for passing still remain a well-guarded secret. The *Bulletin* cites the following generic criteria for evaluation:

1. Develop a diagnosis, including the appropriate clinical, laboratory and diagnostic procedures.
2. Select and apply proper treatment under elective and emergency conditions.
3. Prevent, recognize and manage complications.
4. Plan and direct follow-up and continuing care.

The examination is designed to evaluate your qualifications as a specialist or consultant to non- obstetrician-gynecologist colleagues. The goal of the test is also to evaluate your behavior in independent practice. The emphasis is on patient management knowledge and skills.

The best benchmark or standard to emulate is the ACOG standards. As long as your management is consistent with the ACOG guidelines in the Compendium, you will meet the passing criteria.

The ABOG *Diplomate* publishes the statistics on the exam annually. The pass rate for the oral board exam is higher than for the written board exam; thus, the statistics are much to your favor. Consistently for the last decade, 85% pass the exam on their first attempt.

Your examiners are matched to you based on where you trained and where you currently practice. You are provided this list on the morning of your exam to make sure there are no conflicts of interest.

Recall that you have three pairs of examiners and they will never put two junior examiners together. Each pair does not know who your other examiners are. For example, your obstetric examiners have no idea who is examining you on your office and gynecology sections.

Within a pair, each examiner must grade you for the overall section. Even though an individual examiner will only examine you on half the test, either the case list or the case of the day, he records and observes the conduct of the exam by his co-examiner.

Typically a pair will examine three consecutive candidates. Remember how quickly the next pair of examiners enters upon the hourly chime? The examiners are playing musical chairs. Hopefully, the pair has the opportunity to converse at the end of each three hour session and doesn't have to wait until the end of the day after they've examined six candidates. Each pair must be unanimous in their results. The options are pass, fail, or marginal. Each pair turns in their results independently.

The ABOG *Bulletin* states that the Board of Directors votes on each candidate based on the report of the examining team. Reportedly, a pass is awarded five points, a marginal three points, and a fail one point. You must score ten or more points in order to pass the exam. So do the math yourself. You will pass the exam with the following combinations: 3 pass; 2 pass and one fail or marginal; and 1 pass and two marginal.

The timing of the results suggests that the Board votes at the end of the test week in each of the three months. ABOG insists there is no preplanned pass/fail rate.

ABOG is doing a better job in getting the results to you. In the past, it routinely took six weeks. Now you should have your results in just one week.

Congratulations if you passed! Rest assured—but not for long. The clock starts ticking right away, and soon you must recertify. In 2008, they revamped the recertification process and even gave it a new name, Maintenance of Certification, or MOC. Everyone must complete journal reading along with open book computerized written tests every year. On the sixth year, you must take a written exam. Groan… I know you thought you were over that. Just like GERD, it has come back to haunt you

Traditionally, the recertification written exam was a piece of cake; that is true and is good news if you are a generalist, but bad news for you subspecialists. As you know, you have to maintain your generalist board certification. Everyone must take one of their two test books in general OB/GYN. If you are a generalist, you get to choose your second book. The specialist must take the second book in his subspecialty.

In the unlikely event that you fail your oral board exam, you may repeat it twice—as long as you do so within six years of passing the written exam. After six years, you have to pass the written exam again as you start the cycle over. Effective in 2018, you must achieve basic board certification within 8 years of completing residency. If you have not passed, you will have to complete a minimum of 12 additional months of residency training.

If you Fail…

So… what IF you fail the oral exam? What happens? Well, the easy answer is that you simply retake the exam. The hard answer is preparing you for the maelstrom of emotions that you will experience and need to process in order to be fit to take the exam again. If you are taking the test for the first time, read this chapter once and put it aside. If you fail the test, you must reread this again to understand that you are not alone AND also to learn from others' mistakes.

Back to the easy answer…You may retake the test the next go around. The problem is that it's a bit logistically sticky to pull it off that quickly. Recall that even if you took your test during the first batch of exams, you won't get your results until mid-November. The problem is that case list collections for the test the following year started July 1…or 5 months earlier. This is, of course, even worse if you did not take your exam until January. Talk about being behind the eight ball!

Of course, the shock and realization that you failed takes time to sink in and everybody reacts differently. For those who react by taking the bull by the horns and regaining control, you can pull it off by recapturing the cases quickly. You certainly know what it takes, given you did it just recently. But for those of you immobilized by the dread of starting right back, wait until the following July to start collecting.

Now for the hard answer... As with any major life stress, you will go through the Kubler Ross stages of grief – denial, anger, acceptance and resolution. Many of you will not be surprised that you failed, as you felt like you had already failed when you walked out of the test or especially as you began to ponder your answers. Actually, most have the same feelings, even when they did pass. Unfortunately, that letter from the Executive Director that starts, "Regretfully, I must inform you of your failure to pass the oral board exam..." validates your fear.

One of your toughest chores is having to acknowledge to everyone that you failed. There is no escaping this embarrassing task because anyone who is in any way associated with you knows you've put your whole life on hold for this exam. Unfortunately, you have to inform your spouse, partners, office staff, friends, relatives and the whole world. You feel like there's a billboard in front of your house or office or your forehead is branded with "I failed my oral board exam".

Although you are humiliated and embarrassed, life quickly moves on for others. Think about it – when you hear a rumor or gossip, how long do you linger on it? —Probably only for as long as it took to hear it, right? Do you know any of your colleagues who failed their boards? Do you no longer refer patients to them? Have you ever heard of patients not coming or transferring their care for this reason? The answer is NO! Although this will leave a scar on you, it will not leave even a scratch on anyone else. Life will move on and time softens the blow. You'll know when you're ready to face it again. You must get back in the saddle. Your first task is to figure out, objectively and without emotion, why you failed.

So WHY did you fail? The most common reason cited in that generic letter is "failure to defend your case list". Most admit they simply failed to adequately prepare. The less common reasons are stage fright or exam anxiety or the candidate had no idea. Try to figure out WHY you failed so you can better prepare yourself next time.

Most will acknowledge the "Lessons Learned" noted in Chapter 13. Your strategy next time is simple. You need to prepare both academically and psychologically.

I argue many find the harder of the two is the psychological preparation. You must admit our training in counseling for depression and anxiety is dismal. So why do you feel you are now an authority to get yourself out of this hole? You wouldn't advise your patient to go it alone, so neither should you. You will heal emotionally far quicker if you seek a counselor – a clergy, a psychologist or a psychiatrist. It is a well-known fact that many world-class athletes will seek a sports psychologist. You're no different. He will help you "mind your mind" and help to restore balance.

This time around, keep all the balls in the air, instead of just one. Do not put life on hold – it didn't work before and chances are it won't again. Budget for and embrace personal and family time. A step away from studying rejuvenates the soul and makes you far more effective when you do study.

This time, take the time to develop a study plan as discussed in Chapter 8. Tackle your case list with the vigor and intensity that only a wizened veteran knows how to do. But this time you MUST take mock orals. Almost all who failed admitted they neglected this critical step. Why? Because they viewed this as an acknowledgement of their weakness, rather than as a learning tool. What initially is viewed as a confidence shaker quickly becomes a confidence booster. I promise this is the key to your success next time.

When you retake the exam, the examiners do NOT know that you failed before. You really are at an advantage now, because you DO know what to expect. Make sure you heed that old proverb "trick me once, shame on you; trick me twice, shame on me". Finally, you will learn and grow from this, for "that which does not kill us, will make us stronger".

Chapter 12

A Candidate's Journey

I have been mentoring candidate's preparing for their board exams for nearly twenty five years. Yet it seems like only yesterday when I went through that miserable process myself. Although the blood, sweat, and tears have long dried, I wanted to capture those emotions to help others know what to expect, as forewarned is forearmed.

Everyone's journey is unique, yet we share that same quest to put FACOG behind our beloved MD. I met KJ at our April review course. She was preparing for her oral exams the following fall. I am always impressed with those who have the foresight to be so proactive, as most will delay attending the review course until the fall of the exam. Coincidentally, KJ and I ran into each other at the airport after the course. I knew she was from my state, but discovered she actually practiced only about an hour from me, thus we were on the same flight. Naturally we began to chat.

I applauded her for being ahead in the game. She confessed that actually she was not preparing for the oral exam at all, rather for the written boards *again*. She had failed her written exam and was devastated. "I had *never* failed anything in my life. I was crushed, humiliated, and demoralized. You are actually only the second person I've told. Only my husband knows. I couldn't even tell the rest of my family, friends, nor even my partner".

We physicians are so darn tough on ourselves. But it's true, we don't accept defeat well. Heck, we're devastated if we get a B, but to *fail*? I truly believe that there is no way anyone can make it through four years of college, four years of medical school, and four years of residency if he weren't smart.

161

Can you still practice OB/GYN without being board certified? Yes. But it's not the same without that FACOG behind and lifting up that MD. You know it, I know it, and our colleagues know it. Our patients on the other hand, only understand the MD part.

So this failure, this defeat is a crushing blow. However I have yet to meet a colleague who hasn't acknowledged that picking herself up, facing and overcoming that defeat was one of the most profound growing experiences of her lifetime. KJ was no exception.

We reflected on the past. Turns out she had poorly prepared the first time. She admitted her strength was always as a clinician, not an academician. Her residency did not provide financial, scheduling, academic nor emotional support. She used her vacation time to attend a review course, but her 80- to 100-hour work week did not permit the necessary time to embrace the material.

Well, you usually get out of it, what you put into it. Although she was now very busy in private practice, job #1 was to pass her boards. This time she put her all into it. She passed her written board exam on her second attempt.

She was determined to not make the same mistake twice. Trick me once, shame on you; trick me twice, shame on me. As soon as KJ called me with the good news, I asked her to keep a journal of her journey.

She has attacked preparing for her oral exams with zeal. Although now, you might argue, she's not the typical candidate since she has some baggage, she nonetheless is undertaking this project for the first time. Let's take a peek into her diary.

July 1. "I feel much better about the written exam this time. I really think I did my best. If I failed, it will be hard to figure out what to do differently, but until I know my results, I'm going to proceed full steam ahead. I dug out my ABC (America's OB/GYN Board Review Course) notes. I'm really glad I went to those sessions on case list construction. I didn't so much understand it then, but it was clear that the case list is the biggest player in the exam, and you want to get it right the first time. I recall a lot of complaints about the ABOG software, so I'm going to order the ExamPro software today"

Starting on day 1 of case list collections, KJ started two files; one for Gynecology and the other for Obstetrics. The GYN file contained the admitting history and physical, operative note, discharge summary, pathology report, and office notes for each patient she operated on. The OB file contained the office prenatal record, the admitting history and physical, delivery/operative note, discharge summary, and postpartum visit.

Admittedly, this approach is definitely exploding out of the starting blocks. Because you can't formally apply for the oral exam until February, many will naively not start any work on their case list until then. This is a BIG mistake, as they are already SEVEN MONTHS BEHIND. I think KJ is right on and would strongly recommend you model her record keeping approach.

Also, many erroneously, but innocently assume you must use the ABOG software. This is not true. ABOG mandates only that your list must duplicate exactly their headings. The ABOG software, although much improved over the years, still has some bugs. There are a number of commercial software products that are available too.

August 7 " I got my letter from ABOG today. I was afraid to open it. I held it up to the light. I could see the word "Congratulations," so I tore it open. I PASSED! THANK YOU GOD! I am so glad that's behind me. Life is good. Now I'm pumped up and am going to start entering my cases today"

Good news is a great motivator. I think it is reasonable to wait until you for sure know you passed your written boards before you begin entering your cases. This applies, of course, only for those who chose to take their oral boards immediately after your written boards. If you chose to take a break the year after your written board exam, then there is no excuse to delay. You should have your case list software in hand and start entering cases in July.

September " I am entering my cases weekly. I have the hang of it now. I don't think this artificial intelligence with the ExamPro software is as helpful as I thought it would be. Most of the prompts are self explanatory. Funny how you don't have any control about the type of cases. I find with every patient I see, wondering how it's going to play out on my case list."

October " I got my passport pictures taken today for my application. I told Paul [her husband] I felt like I was getting my mug shot taken for prison. Case list collections are going well. I find it's easier to just enter them at the end of the day. I know I'm probably adding way too much information, but I figure I can always delete extraneous information later"

I agree that it's better to initially front load by entering too much information on your case list. You can later unload ballast. However if you are later needing to fill in with missing detail, then it's tedious and wastes time to backtrack.

November "Well, I sent my application in today. It felt good to formally get the ball rolling. I can't believe it's so expensive to just apply. I'm going to have to deal out another $900 just for the examination fee. Oh well, it sure beats the alternative."

January 6 " I met with Dr. Das today, just to make sure I'm on track since I'm at the half way mark. I figure it will be easier to fix problems now. She made me look at the list in a way I never even thought of, that is from the *examiner's* perspective. Gee, why didn't I think of that? It makes sense. It's far more logical to word the cases *before submission* to strategically control the questions that I want **them** to ask me.

"She also showed me her case list library. These are binders filled with case lists. She very quickly convinced me how the *physical appearance* of a case list makes a huge impression. When you have the luxury to look at a big stack of case lists, I realized the outstanding ones were obvious within seconds. Of course, my only perspective until then was my own."

"She showed me some of her favorites; these were obviously customized. She told me that one of them was created by the teenage son of a candidate. Several others she claimed were drafted in the evenings of the review course. Could it really be *that easy*? I've got 6 months left. I don't want to have one of those cookie cutter case lists. I want to stand out. I'm going to create her new favorite"

Note KJ deliberately did not start with the ABOG case list software. However she discovered the commercial software did not meet her expectations either. Sometimes you have to appreciate what you don't like, to help you better define what you do want. She has plenty of time to transition to a different program.

January 12 "I have been working with Debbie (ABC's Operations Manager and a "computer genius" according to Dr. Das) by e-mail, but today we met. I showed her how I created my custom case list with Microsoft Word using tables. She had recommended Excel spreadsheets, but she likes my idea. Admittedly, my timing for this project was lousy, since I upgraded my computer. It's difficult to create a case list, learn about something in Microsoft that I have never used before *and* figure out the new computer all at once. This would be horrible if it was June and the deadline was quickly approaching!"

Amen to the not putting if off until the end! KJ had the luxury to work with Debbie. Obviously she was able to meet with her since she was geographically close. In this day and age; however, you can easily obtain a consult by tele-conference, videoconference, e-mail etc. There are also case list construction workshops that are available starting in the spring. Interesting that KJ, through experimentation on her own, was able to present a new way, even to a seasoned veteran.

February "My spiffy new case list is polished and much better organized. Reentering the cases was very good because it made me rethink the cases. I threw out details that were not important and added ones that I missed previously. Dr. Das will not have to use much of that red ink next time, that I'm sure!"

Chapter 12 • A Candidate's Journey

March "Began to collect my office cases. I gave Kristie [her medical assistant] a list of the office practice categories. She is really taking it to heart. She'll whisper in my ear, "this would be a good one for your case list"."

April "Pulled out my ABC case list construction notes and reread Dr. Das' book. I'm starting to shift cases and reword [the notes], trying to put in some strategy. Starting to pull references for topics".

By this time, you get routed into a habit. It's good to revisit the whole issue, as now you are able to appreciate hints and tips that you glossed over earlier. This is definitely a fluid process. If you haven't already, this is a good time to invest in a case list construction workshop.

May 20 " Met with Dr. Das and we reviewed my OB and Office case list. Does this lady ever run out of red ink??! Discovered I have bullet toxicity (no, not the one from the gun, but after that session, doesn't sound like a bad alternative). Learned bullets for the OB are a completely different organizational tool than for the GYN case list. Decided to put that project on hold until after Army Reserve Annual Training. I'll prioritize getting the Office collections done and be up to date on OB and GYN collections."

Ideally you need to have your case list reviewed for construction tips about this time. This gives you plenty of time to deliberately put/word cases exactly to meet your strategic objective.

June " Met one last time with Dr. Das. My case list is just about ready to go. There is very little red ink this time. I am having some formatting challenges but for the most part I am satisfied with the outcome. I feel sorry for those who waited until the last minute and are fighting with their office staff and medical records for data. I am glad I started this process early. And I'm glad I had a mentor in this process. I can't imagine doing it alone."

July 3 "Received letter from ABOG that my application has been accepted. I also was surprised they said my exam is in January. Gosh, they haven't even received my case list, yet I already have my exam date… or at least the month of my exam. I have mixed emotions. I wish it was in November, then I would be done with it earlier, but then again, it will give me more time to prepare."

July. "I'm pleased with my second draft. It really paid off to work so hard earlier, because it's so easy to make the changes now. It's going to be weird not working on this anymore. I feel like it's part of my daily routine. I'm doing fine on time"

July 23 "Sent my case list—taking NO chances of UPS losing it. I have my tracking number and sent it signature request receipt so ABOG has to verify they received it. Boy do I feel like a huge weight has been lifted off my shoulders. I have no regrets with how I constructed that list."

August, September "Since my exam is not until January, I've gone fishin'. I'm going to play, have fun, and *not* think about the boards or that case list at all"

June and July is all consuming with finishing the case list. It's a good idea to take a break. If your exam is in November, then you can't step away as long as those whose exam is in January.

October 21 "I went to ABC's Oral Exam Workshop … talk about an eye opener. We were paired up and reviewed each others case list. You could tell some were just thrown together with little thought. Some people left themselves wide open for questions about topics that no one wants to discuss. Some lists were boring with "AUB" over and over again and the same management every time. Some people did not follow directions about the number of cases on the office list (40) or about making the lists HIPPA compliant. I felt very good about my case list and now know that it was well worth the time and effort that I put into it.

"On the other hand, I need to study! During the workshop, I volunteered to be in the hot seat and the other candidates quizzed me. I could answer some of their questions, but I could tell that most of them had been studying while I was goofing off in August and September. No more break for me! Now I'm ready to focus during the Review Course for the next five days".

October 22-26 "I attended the ABC Board Review Course. During that time, I made a study plan. Some of the topics I knew well, but it seems like l learned new things even during those lectures. Throughout the course I made a list of one-liners, things I had always meant to learn/memorize but never seemed to have the time, to study later. I highlighted some things in the syllabus during the lectures, but because my focus is more clinical this time, I spent more time *listening* rather than just writing down every word. The speakers were excellent so I actually enjoyed listening too. I especially liked how exam focused they were, so it helps me focus my studying.

"We "oral exam takers" gave each other mock oral exams about the lectures during the breaks. One of my favorite parts about the course was meeting people like me who were as panicked. We met in the evenings to study too because a few had to sit for their boards in less than two weeks. I'm glad that's not me, but on the other hand, I wish it was."

November 7 "Met with Dr. Das to just strategize what to do from now until my exam. I told her I'm going to take a few weeks off over the holidays and really focus on studying without my cell phone or patient responsibilities. Paul and I are going back home and travel for two weeks over Christmas.

We get back on Sunday, January 4. I have explained to Paul that I won't be able to socialize because I have to study. Dr. Das has insisted that I spend some quality time with family without guilt about not studying. It is very hard to find balance. Still haven't heard the exact date of my exam, but worse case scenario, if it's the Monday, then I'll have 8 days left. Dr. Das suggested we schedule a mock oral in December before I leave and then immediately upon my return. Damn, now I'm starting to get nervous. Maybe I shouldn't have blown off studying in August and September. It's too late to cancel my trip and Paul would kill me. OK, not to panic. I can do this.

I am studying for about two hours a day and 6-8 hours on the weekends. I am actually enjoying it quite a bit since this is about my patients. Previous studying has been to answer a specific question. This time I am studying to have a discussion about a patient. This is what I do everyday when someone "curbsides" me about a patient or when I discuss patients with colleagues. In my day to day conversations with my partners I am practicing for my oral boards."

December 7 "Took the day off yesterday to spend time with family and today I am studying. Meeting with MFM for mock oral Dec 9 after work. I am going to review my OB notes and case list before the meeting so I can be prepared. This will be my first mock oral so I don't really know how I am going to do but I'm not too nervous because I discuss patients with her pretty regularly."

December 8 "Spoke with local REI and he has agreed to meet with me in January. He even offered to buy dinner because he knows what I'm going through. I got my letter with the date for my oral exam. Last day, last session. I guess I get more time to prepare than almost everyone else taking the boards. I'm not sure if this is good or bad. More time to worry too."

"I called the local hotels for reservations but a lot of them are sold out. A couple people have advised me not to stay at the Melrose because it is pretty noisy and difficult to sleep. I don't think I'll be sleeping much at that point anyway, but I'll take their advice. Made reservations to arrive on Jan 14 for my Jan 16 exam. That should give me a little quiet time away from my cell phone, office and family responsibilities."

December 10 "I met with the MFM for a case list review and mock oral last night. She gave me some really good pointers. She advised me to always repeat the question because it gives time to think and to only answer the question asked. This makes sense to me. She pulled some topics out of my case list that she is pretty sure the examiners will ask. She didn't really ask me any questions and I didn't ask her to because I was afraid that I wouldn't know the answers. Ugh! Isn't that why I asked for this meeting. Isn't it better to be miserable now so that I won't be as miserable later????"

You need to give your mock oral examiner guidance on how to conduct the session if they have no experience. Refer back to Chapter 8 for that list. Although volume is helpful, the more mock oral exams, the better; it's even more helpful if you get a quality exam. Remember *perfect practice* makes perfect.

December 16 *&^**!#! Met with Dr. Das last night for mock orals. MISERABLE!!! She really knows how to find the little things that I don't know and magnify them. Who cares about "mechanism of action"? I know it works and how to use it. I need to go home and hi-light all the drugs on my case list and memorize the MOA's so the examiners won't be able to make me as miserable as she has. I guess I don't have much of a poker face because she could tell every time the questions she asked were out of my comfort zone. I need to learn to relax and not tense up and start stuttering when I don't know the answer to a question right away. I will be sooooo happy when this whole process is over! I know how to take care of patients and this is very frustrating!

"I still haven't done any Christmas shopping, sent any cards or attended a party. It seems like all I do is study and work. I can't wait for my vacation next week. I know I can get some real studying done if I get out of town and away from my cell phone."

December 26 "Landed in Frankfurt, Germany today. I reviewed all of the GYN sections of my notes in the airport and on the flight. I got a lecture from Paul about ruining the trip by studying too much, but we discussed this before we made the reservation. I have promised to spend some free time with him but my goal is to focus on studying for the boards. "

December 27 "It was a great day today strolling from one café to another. Coffee and amenorrhea...Hot chocolate and the new Pap guidelines...chocolate and postpartum hemorrhage... I hope I can still fit into my suit when I get home."

Regardless of when your exam is, at least one, if not both of your holidays are ruined. By this time, studying and the looming exam are heavy on your mind. Remember to at least budget time off and stick to it! You will feel less guilty, your family will be appreciative, and your studying will be more focused.

December 30 "OK now I am stressing out. I should have finished the first review of all the notes by now. I only have 3 weeks to go and we are heading to see family today. How am I going to get everything memorized in time? Maybe I should have stayed home."

Chapter 12 • A Candidate's Journey

You will always feel like you can study more. There will always be some items left over on your study list.

January 1 "I haven't studied in 2 days. I keep thinking about how Dr. Das said to spend some quality time away from my studies and enjoy my family. I needed a break but now I'm ready to buckle down again. How would I possibly do this if I had kids? My friends set up a little office for me complete with drinks, snacks and Internet. I feel guilty studying instead of visiting but we told everyone about my "important test" before we made the reservations. Everyone is wishing me luck and praying for me to pass. How miserable is it going to be if I don't pass? This pressure is all consuming. Everyone at the hospital knows. Everyone at my office knows. What if I don't pass? How will I face everyone? "

January 7 "Back to the good old USA. I am back on track and on schedule. I met with my local REI for a mock oral on my office case list. We went one case at a time and he quizzed me for 3 hours. At 3 different times he told me I was going to pass. Yeah! My studying is paying off. This was a little too easy. I hope the examiners are as reasonable as he was."

January 8 "Another mock oral and structured cases with Dr. Das. I don't know how she does it, but she can find the little things that you thought you knew but obviously didn't know well enough. She busted me again on those stupid MOA's. This no feedback thing is tough. How do you know if you are answering the questions correctly? It's no wonder when most people leave the exam they think they've failed. I sure hope I don't feel that way. Too many people are counting on me to pass."

January 13 "I think I'm gonna throw up! My husband said good bye and good luck to me this morning and could feel the tears welling up. What if I don't pass? I don't want to have that conversation "I know you did your best…Those stupid people don't know anything…You are the best doctor I know…" What if I start crying when the examiner asks me something I don't know? What if I just sit there and can't think? What if I forget the mechanism of action of methotrexate? Can they fail you for that? What if I don't pass? How humiliating!

"This pressure is all consuming and not worth it! I wonder if there is someone else as stressed out about this stupid process as I am. Maybe I'm crazy. I know I must have studied enough to pass but what if the examiners can find my weaknesses as easily as Dr. Das can? I had my colleagues quiz me and I knew almost all of the answers to their questions. My studying has definitely made me more confident with them. I know a lot. I know enough to pass. I WILL PASS!!!

January 13 "My flight leaves at 7AM, so I'm staying at a hotel by the airport. Dr. Das came for one last hoorah session. I was hoping to bribe her with desert, as I've figured out she usually softens with this tactic. She just got back from Dallas last night giving ABC's mock oral exams just before the test. She's been in the office all day, then a dinner meeting and unfortunate for me, already had desert. She looked tired, but seemed to really perk up at the thought of torturing me with my final mock oral.

"Reviewed vaginal breech, TVT vs TOT and more. I know a lot more now than I did the last time we got together. However she managed to pull out a drug that wasn't even on my case list. That's simply not fair. I had told her after our last encounter that I was going to learn all the MOAs for each drug on my case list. So she demanded to quiz me on my drug cards. She tried to bore right through me, but I stood my ground. After going through half the deck, she conceded and retreated, and acknowledged I knew them well. HAH!! One for ME, and a big fat zero for Das. I'm ready, let me at 'em.

"She told me that I deserve to pass. I know I must deserve to pass but I'm not perfect and neither is my knowledge base. I have a little more to study over the next few days but she says it's too late to learn and I think she's right. I need to relax. I can't remember if I know how to do that."

The week of the exam is the toughest. What's done is done. Nothing more to do. You can't possibly learn anything more, and that reality just hits you squarely in your face. Now you have to accept that you have no more control ...and that's depressing and terrifying. There is no turning back. You've waited so long for this week, yet it is suddenly here. You must get yourself psyched up. ONLY *positive* thoughts. I WILL PASS. I think I can. No, I KNOW I can. Yay me!!"

January 14 "Arrived in Dallas without a hitch. There's a blizzard in Chicago. I hope those people gave themselves a little buffer. I doubt ABOG will be too sympathetic about acts of nature. I'm sure they would be happy to let those folk come back next year no charge.

"I am staying at a Marriott hotel because I heard the Melrose was too noisy to study [in]. I need time away from everything and time to breathe, to focus and to figure out how not to freeze when the questions start. I think I am hypercritical of myself because I know the pain of failure. I don't want that to happen again. This is a very emotional time for me and I can't freak myself out thinking about it too much. I made reservations for a massage and facial tomorrow. Reviewed a few things before bed but nothing is sticking in my brain anymore."

It's a good idea to arrive one or two days before. The winter weather is so unpredictable, and it's risky to have no wiggle room in case of delays. If you will have a time zone change, then you need time to acclimate. There are pros/cons at staying at the Melrose, which is where you meet the day of the test. Some want to be in that environment and own it! Others want to avoid it like the plague. What is your strategy? Get a good night sleep tonight, but the night before your exam will be restless.

January 15 DAY BEFORE "Aaaaahhh! Leisurely breakfast…massage with Gabriel, facial with Leslie…Now I'm ready. One more quick look at my notes because I feel obligated. I wonder what the other applicants are doing now. Probably cramming. 24 hours from now and it will all be over. I won't put myself through this process again. Too much pressure! I hope I pass. I hope I can sleep tonight. I'm glad I'm not staying at the noisy Melrose."

Try and relax. Do whatever it takes. Treat yourself. You deserve it. No studying.

January 16 EXAM DAY 0300 (3AM) "Test day. Can't sleep. The bed is comfortable and the room is quiet, but I'm getting excited. I'm ready. I know I'm ready. I wish I were in the morning group. I should try to get some more sleep or I'll be feeling my usual sleepiness in the afternoon. I definitely won't be having coffee with lunch because we won't get a bathroom break for 3 hours. I'm a little nervous about that. Even if I have to go, I'll hold it so the wrong answers I give will count for less. Hmmm…If I am doing well and they ask something I don't know should I then ask for a bathroom break?? I'm over-thinking again. I'm going back to bed."

January 16 EXAM DAY 1000 (10:00AM) "Ok, so I've said my final good byes to everyone and I have prayers and brainwaves coming from every direction and I'm freaking out. I have no good reason to freak out and I'm freaking out. I am so afraid of failure it hurts. Dr. Das just sent a text message "Remember just 70%." I love this woman. She absolutely knows what to say to ease your mind. I don't have to be perfect. Just 70%. Time to get dressed and stop crying. I'm such a baby. If my referring docs could only see me now!"

January 16 EXAM DAY 1030 (10:30AM) "I look sharp! This suit is great. The shoes are good. My hair is just right. I'm gonna knock 'em dead!!! Caselist, ID, no cell phone. I'm outta here. The next time I see this room I'll be finished with the boards!"

January 16 EXAM DAY 1700 (5PM) "It was definitely an exhausting day. I really felt like they try to make it even more dramatic than it needed to be with all of the procedural stuff. They give you a time to be at the conference room at the hotel, and then have you all sit in this room with a bunch of stressed people in suits waiting until the specified time. Then instead of registering you as you came in, they call you up front to register in groups of two. It really just dragged the whole process and made everyone even more nervous!

"I'm 90% sure I passed but I'm 100% done. Yahoo!!! That wasn't too bad. I heard stories from others that they had really tough examiners but mine were reasonable. It was tough when they grabbed on to something I wasn't sure about, but that's my fault.

"The things I didn't know were things I would have never considered studying or were things I had reviewed but just forgot at the moment. There were a lot of differential diagnosis questions, especially in the case of the day questions. I really thought the case list questions were straightforward and easy- because I knew my case list well. I thought that was easier than the case of the days simply because I knew what to expect and was more prepared for those questions.

"I'm a good doctor. I am a good obstetrician and gynecologist. I may not know it all but I know how to find the answers when I need them. If I don't pass this test, I don't know what else I could possibly do to better prepare. I passed. I'm sure of it. But I don't want to jinx it so I'll say 90%. Time to celebrate being done!!!!

January 17 Day After "Woke up with a headache this morning. I am trying not to think about the test too much, but I keep thinking of things I may have answered incorrectly. They asked about a 40- weeker with a precipitous delivery of an 1800g baby. All I could think of was the differential diagnosis for IUGR and we talked about that for a while. I think they really wanted to know about resuscitation, but I didn't figure that out until about 4am. Oh jeez! This is torture!"

January 21 "I dreamed last night that I opened the envelope and it said "We are sorry to inform you…" I woke up VERY relieved that it was only a dream. I have been trying to keep busy so I don't have time to think about it but the wait is killing me."

January 22, 2009 "I got a call from Dr. Das this afternoon that a guy in Virginia got his scores today. Now I'm afraid to go home and check the mail. I won't let Paul check because I don't want him to have to think of a way to let me down gently. I was 90% sure I passed but now I'm only 70% sure. Part of me wants to hurry home but part of me hopes that I don't get the letter today. If it doesn't come I can still be 70% sure I passed instead of 0%."

January 23, 2009 11:00am "No mail yesterday. I saw patients this morning and made my office manager cancel my afternoon meeting with my accountant. If I fail, I won't be able to pay attention and if I pass I won't be able to pay attention. My sister says the mailman comes between 11:30 and 11:45am while I'm at work. She knows this because she waits for him often. She even knows his name and all about his children. Maybe I should ask her to put in a good word for me. Everyone in the office knows I'm going home to check the mail. If I fail I am not going to get out of bed this weekend and I might stay in bed next week too. I will be "certified nuts" if not board certified. UGGGhhhh....this waiting is awful! "

January 23, 2009 11:45am "YAHOO!!!!!! I PASSED!!!!!!!! OMG I CAN'T BELIEVE IT!!! YES I CAN!!!!! I KNEW I WOULD PASS!!!!!!!!

I carried the envelope from the mailbox into the kitchen because I was afraid to see what was inside. I opened it with Paul and I saw the word "Congratulations!" That's all it took to make me start sobbing like a baby. Paul kept saying "No, it's okay, YOU PASSED!!!" I had no idea what the rest of the letter said but the first word was "Congratulations!" You know me… I started thinking… I wonder if it says "Congratulations… you failed and get to start the whole wonderful process over again!" I made Paul read the whole letter to me but I didn't really hear what he was saying after the first few lines. I started calling and texting everyone I know starting with Dr Das. No one knows how much this test meant to me more than her. It felt so good to have the people that mean so much to me texting back their congratulations. One of my friends even shouted out the good news to everyone in the hospital cafeteria! Another asked if she could put it on her Facebook page because she was so proud of me."

Afterthoughts: "If I had it to do all over again (WHICH I DON'T!!!) I would do everything the same way. I am very lucky to have failed my written boards the first time. That might sound crazy but I didn't know what I didn't know. What I mean is failing made me truly embrace the learning process.

"In residency I was groomed to believe that I knew more than my peers because of our powerhouse program. That was not true. I am a very good and capable surgeon but my academic skills were lacking because no one expressed to me the importance of academics. Sure, I learned all about specialized research and how to care for the zebras but I missed out on a lot of the basics. Like most of us, I had never failed anything before in my life. It was devastating to get the letter telling me I was a failure at what I had just spent 120hrs a week for the last four years doing. It didn't really say I was a failure but that's what it felt like. I was devastated and humiliated and I told **no one** except for my husband and later Dr. Das.

"After I picked myself up, I vowed to study like I was in medical school again and I did. I took Dr. Das' ABC course and memorized everything in the huge binder. I could even quote the ACOG *Compendium*. I passed my written board exam on the second try and I passed as a much better physician, not only a good clinician but a good academician.

"I started this journal just after I passed the written exam and I studied for another 18 months. This time I studied while I cared for my patients. Because the oral exam is all about how you function as you care for your patients, I actually enjoyed the process. There was a lot of stress for me because of the previous failure, and all the emotions that that created, but I think that has made passing the oral exam that much sweeter.

"You won't find a mentor more passionate about her job than Dr. Das. She went far above and beyond my expectations because she genuinely cares. I think she feels responsible for making sure all of her protégé succeed and this is what makes her stand out among her peers. If you think you can't do it, call her. If you need to relearn the basics, sign up for an ABC course. Go early in the year to give yourself time to study. Get help with case list construction so you have a better chance of discussing topics **you** want to discuss rather than those you don't. Put yourself through mock orals with anyone who will talk to you and if you can, make an early reservation to have Dr. Das or one of her ABC staff torture you too. There was almost nothing that the examiners asked me that I hadn't heard before either at the ABC course or one-one one with Dr. Das.

"Good Luck!"

—KJ, MD, FACOG

Chapter 13

Lessons Learned

After the exam is over and the dust has settled (or perhaps more appropriately, after the blood, sweat, and tears have dried), I have asked candidates, "If you had to do it all over again, what would you do differently?" Below are the most frequent responses.

1. **Start collecting my case list earlier and updating it more frequently (regularly).**

   Recommendation: Start collecting cases on July 1 and enter them after every surgery and delivery.

   Start collecting cases on July 1. Begin collecting and entering your gynecologic cases after every surgery, and your obstetric cases after every delivery. Put some blank case list forms in your locker in Labor and Delivery and Surgery, in your office and in your briefcase. Better yet, put a form in the patient's office chart when you head over to surgery and fill it out in the operating room after you dictate the procedure. Match these rough drafts with the accompanying history and physical, operative or delivery notes and discharge summary.

   If you cannot update after every surgery or delivery, do so *at least weekly*. If you procrastinate more than two weeks, you will have lost recall of precious details. In the long term, you will waste more time, and experience more frustration in trying to capture lost dates and details.

   For the office case list collection, I recommend you keep a list of the categories on your desk starting in August. Over the next few months, simply jot down the patient's name and diagnosis when they fit a particular category. Once you have four names in a category, cease further collection.

Every two to three months, pull the corresponding office chart and develop a rough draft case list for each one. At the 5- to 6-month mark, begin an earnest search for those hard-to-find categories. In April, select your final 40 patients.

2. I would not use the ABOG computer program for case list collection.

Recommendation: Initially, use the ABOG case list software, but convert to a custom list in January.

Most candidates innocently, but mistakenly assume they *must* use the ABOG program. This is *not* true! This misperception is further propagated because your application acceptance letter "strongly suggests" that you purchase the ABOG case list software, claiming that "some commercially available programs do not print an acceptable case list". However, the ABOG *Bulletin* specifies that you only need to duplicate the *format* of the example case list forms. The ABOG program improves with each edition, but it is still fraught with frustrating software glitches. Worse yet, you have little control over the order of patients, categories and procedures. These are key strategical elements.

I recommend you construct *your own* program. Appendix D contains some tips. Not only are you in complete control of the best way to implement your strategy, but you can also optimize presentation and organization. Your case list will be a one-of-a-kind and not a cookie-cutter duplication of those who used the ABOG or commercial software.

However, you don't have the best feel for what you want from your case list until you get the basics down. Thus, I recommend you *start* with the ABOG software. You can order it from the ABOG web site at **www.ABOG.org**. Don't worry which edition you purchase, as you will convert later. You can even borrow one of your colleague's programs from last year, as often the edition for your year isn't available until the fall. Do not delay until this edition is available, as you will be too far backlogged. I recommend you start entering cases no later than (NLT) September.

After a few months, you will quickly understand your predecessor's grumbles. That's good, because now you know what you *don't want*. Ideally, design your custom case list in January or February. You can wait as late as May because, believe it or not, this can be accomplished in just a few hours. Help is available for technical support from the consultants listed in Appendix D.

Remember, your examiners review your case list *before* they examine you. Your case list is your DNA of the way you manage patients. The examiner's *first impression* of you is based on your case list. The money is clearly in the case list! Take the time to do it right.

3. I would have had my case list reviewed *before* I submitted it August 1.

Recommendation: In May or June, have your case list reviewed for construction advice.

After August 1, your case list is set in stone. Only later, when you begin preparing for its defense, do you sorrowfully appreciate how much easier it would be if you had only reworded the case.

I recommend tapping into your colleagues' collective wisdom. I would use local, regional and academic clinicians, as well as both generalists and subspecialists. Their job is to give their recommendations on how to word each case. Only you know what your strategic objective is with each case and to then come up with the final wording. Chances are neither you nor your consultants have had much experience in constructing case lists. It is well-worth your money to have a seasoned professional review your last draft, to help you masterfully add the finishing touches to the masterpiece.

I forewarn that you must be organized and disciplined to pull this off. Send whatever you have of your case list to your colleagues in early May, with the deadline to have it back to you mid-May. You then need to send it to the professional consultant by early June. This will give you time for only one major rewrite before you must send it in to meet the August 1 deadline.

4. I would have started studying earlier.

Recommendation: Start intense studying by mid-August.

These are the famous last words of all students. Remember, it has been a while since you had to buckle down and *really* study. The last time was when you were preparing for the written boards. Not only are you out of shape, but probably you have never prepared for an oral exam. It is *not* the same as a written exam.

Chapter 4, *Getting Started*, contains tips on how to budget your time and Chapter 8, *Studying for the Exam*, suggests strategies for studying. Your priority before August 1 is that darn case list. However, if you have a November test date, you really need to come out breathing fire by mid-August. If your test is later, you have a little wiggle room, but don't get lax and let precious study time dwindle away.

The bottom line: "To thine own self be true." Don't kid yourself—do an honest appraisal of what is practical, especially given your time constraints. To quote Nike—"Just do it!"

5. I would not have studied the pathology slides.

Recommendation: Don't study microscopic pathology.

Interpretation of gross and microscopic pathology is no longer a distinct exam component. If a Kodachrome is shown, it most likely will be labeled with the diagnosis. If it is not, you do not lose points for not knowing the diagnosis. What is important is your ability to apply your clinical acumen in *managing* the patient with the disease. I wouldn't study *any* microscopic slides. If you feel compelled to do so, review mucinous and serous cystadenocarcinoma of the ovary and endometrial hyperplasia and carcinoma. If you are ridiculously compulsive and want to eat up precious time, study the 27 slides listed in Table 3 of Chapter 8.

6. I would have had my case list reviewed *after* I submitted it August 1.

Recommendation: Have your case list reviewed for potential questions in August.

Now that your case list is set in stone, you must defend it. You and the consultants discussed in #3 must view your case list from the examiner's eyes and predict what kind of questions he will ask. The more sets of eyes that review your list, the more overlap. Also, you will see a clear pattern emerging and will be able to narrow down the top ten cases. Predicting your test topics will enable you to prioritize your studying, as well as focus your mock oral exams.

7. I should have taken a *board* review course

Recommendation: Take a board review course in the spring and/or the fall.

Time is precious and tight. It seems like it was easier to find the time when you were a resident. Now everybody wants your time – family, practice, church, etc. Take the time to research the various review courses available. I recommend you find a *board* review course, which is targeted specifically to preparing you for your board exam, rather than just a general review. Take into consideration how long the course is and how long you will be away from the office. Chapter 4 can help guide you.

Bottom line: you must step away. Few can review the volume and intensity of subjects on their own. You will be much more efficient by going to a review course. Make sure however, that they streamline and focus your studying to high yield exam topics.

8. **I should have attended a tutorial workshop**

   Recommendation: In the spring, attend a workshop on Case List Construction and in the fall, attend one on Oral Exam Conduct and Strategy.

   Strategy and tactics is involved throughout the entire process. Why reinvent the wheel when you can tap into others' collective wisdom? I recommend you take a one day workshop on how to construct your case list. This will not only give you specific ideas to incorporate, but also get a number of pairs of eyes on your cases. You will exponentially advance in getting to a polished product, while giving up only one day. I recommend attending only after you have some experience under your belt in working with your case list. Thus, I suggest you attend in late winter or spring, so you have time to incorporate the strategy.

   Along that same theme, if you've never taken your oral board exam, why take chances? Again, tap into those who have mentored many and have the expertise and feedback to give you timely tips and help. I recommend attending a one or two day workshop on oral exam strategy within one or two months of your exam.

9. **I would have taken (more) mock oral exams.**

   Recommendation: Take at least three mock orals, starting NLT one month before your exam. Have at least one of them administered by a professional and/or subspecialist.

   The learning curve for taking an oral exam is no different than any other exponential learning curve for a new skill. When you first learned to tie surgical knots, you had to practice. This is no different, and actually a lot easier.

   Most candidates can get to the top of the learning curve with just *three* mock orals. A pool of examiners is right at your fingertips. Just pick up the phone and call your referring MFM, oncologist or REI. Even easier, call one of your local generalist colleagues. Have him or her review your case list to identify test topics. After you have studied your case list, ask him or her to give you a mock oral.

You need to get your first mock oral under your belt no later than one month before your exam. Obviously, you need to get the remaining two within the one to two weeks before the test. You definitely need to take at least one with someone who does not know you; this strips away any "home-court" bias. I recommend a faculty member at one of the review courses or a colleague of one of your referral consultants.

10. I would have started collecting my Chief year cases sooner.

Recommendation: If you plan to limit your practice (Laborist, GYN-only, etc.) or subspecialize, begin collecting cases in your off-specialty at the beginning of your senior year of residency.

Life is unpredictable. How many knew you would end up exactly where you are today? I know it sounds crazy, but you might get an insane notion and decide to do a subspecialty fellowship or limit your practice. Thus, my recommendation for ALL residents… **Hold onto your chief residency case log!** Once you know you really will be going on to a fellowship, then begin collecting cases from your Chief year in your non-fellowship discipline. Unless you stay in the same town as your residency, it is a nightmare to go back and collect cases. I recommend you begin collecting cases just as I recommended for Lessons Learned #1. Do not put off until tomorrow what you can do today!

11. I would have taken the basic oral exam earlier in my fellowship.

Recommendation: Apply for your basic oral exam the first year of your fellowship.

Prior to 2013, subspecialty fellows were not even allowed to sit for their basic oral exam until the second year of their fellowship. However, you can now take it anytime. Of course, not all fellowship directors are in full support of this and may discourage you from taking it until the third research year. You will quickly forget those off specialty topics. The longer you wait, the worse the recall. You need to persuade him that it's to the program's advantage for you to take the exam as soon as possible, as this will enhance your chances of passing. Remind him that you cannot sit for your subspecialty oral exam until after you have passed your basic oral exam. You want to assure your program's reputation.

If you're no longer practicing general OB/GYN, you peaked in your chief residency year. You can't imagine forgetting how to deliver a baby or performing a hysterectomy, since you can practically do it in your sleep.

But truly, if you don't use it, you'll lose it. The candidate who can readily tap into their everyday clinical practice during the exam is at an advantage. See if you can staff the resident clinic or take call for ED and L&D, so you can enhance your retention. Apply for your basic oral exam during the first year of your fellowship. Recall even this means the earliest that you will be sitting for the exam will not be until fall of your second year, since you had to collect cases the first year of your fellowship.

Appendix A

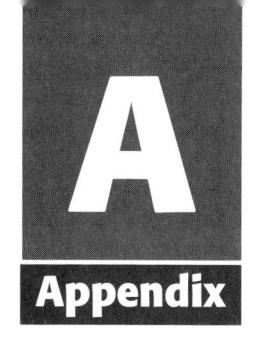

ABOG Acceptable Case List Abbreviations

Check the ABOG Bulletin for the most up-to-date list of approved abbreviations, but don't feel like you have to limit yourself to only these abbreviations. I am not aware of any case list being rejected for using a few that are not on this list—just use conventional abbreviations. The columns are narrow and your case list gets cluttered with tedious long words that are conventionally abbreviated. For example, I would use DMPA rather than spelling out Depo Medroxyprogesterone Acetate. Avoid regional colloquialisms such as IOL, Induction of Labor. An easy check to make sure your abbreviation is conventional and not regional, is to take your case list to the review course and get a couple of opinions from a few folks who are not geographically close. If everyone instantly recognizes and uses the same abbreviation, then I would use that abbreviation.

Do not amend the ABOG abbreviations. For example, I would suggest not using NSVD, normal spontaneous vaginal delivery, in lieu of the ABOG recommended abbreviation of SVD, spontaneous vaginal delivery. Admittedly, some of their abbreviations are atypical: for example, CD for cesarean delivery rather than C/S for cesarean section. However, when in Rome, do as the Romans.

A&P repair	Anterior and posterior colporrhaphy
AB	Abortion
AIDS	Acquired immune deficiency syndrome
ASCUS	Atypical cells of undetermined significance
BSO	Bilateral salpingo-oophorectomy
BTL	Bilateral tubal ligation
CBC	Complete blood count
CD	Cesarean delivery
CIN	Cervical intraepithelial neoplasia
cm	Centimeter
CT	Computerized tomography
D&C	Dilatation and curettage
D&E	Dilatation and evacuation
DEXA	Dual-energy x-ray absorptiometry
DHEAS	Dehydroepiandrosterone sulfate

DVT	Deep venous thrombosis
E	Estrogen
E2	Estradiol
EKG/ECG	Electrocardiogram
FSH	Follicle-stimulating hormone
GDM	Gestational diabetes mellitus
gms	Grams
HIV	Human immunodeficiency virus
HCG	Human chorionic gonadotropin
HPV	Human papillomavirus
HRT	Hormone replacement therapy
HSV	Herpes simplex virus
IM	Intramuscular
IUD	Intrauterine device
IUGR	Intrauterine growth restriction
IV	Intravenous
kg	Kilogram
LAVH	Laparoscopic assisted vaginal hysterectomy
LEEP	Loop electrosurgical procedure
LH	Luteinizing hormone
MRI	Magnetic resonance imaging
P	Progesterone
PAP	Papanicolaou smear
PPH	Postpartum hemorrhage
PROM	Premature rupture of membranes
PTL	Preterm labor
SAB	Spontaneous abortion
SROM	Spontaneous rupture of membranes
STD/STI	Sexually transmitted disease/infection
SVD	Spontaneous vaginal delivery
T	Testosterone
TAH	Total abdominal hysterectomy
TSH	Thyroid-stimulating hormone
TVH	Total vaginal hysterectomy
VBAC	Vaginal birth after cesarean delivery

Appendix B

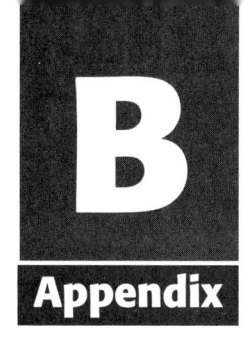

Acronyms and Abbreviations

ABC	America's OB/GYN Board Review Course
A&P	Anterior and posterior colporrhaphy
ABOG	American Board of Obstetrics and Gynecology, Inc.
ACOG	American College of Obstetricians and Gynecologists
AUB	Abnormal uterine bleeding
BHCG	Beta human chorionic gonadotropin
BSO	Bilateral salpingo-oophorectomy
CD	Cesarean delivery
CIN	Cervical intraepithelial neoplasia
CMS	Center for Medicare and Medicaid Services
c/o	Complains of
CREOG	Council on Resident Education in Obstetrics and Gynecology
CS	Cesarean section
CT	Computerized tomography
D&C	Dilatation and curettage
DIC	Disseminated intravascular coagulation
DMPA	Depo Medroxyprogesterone acetate
EGA	Estimated gestational age
EKG	Electrocardiogram
FACOG	Fellow of the American College of Obstetrians and Gynecologists
FPM/FPMRS	Female Pelvic Medicine & Reconstructive Surgery
G	Gravida
GDM	Gestational Diabetes Mellitus
GnRH	Gonadotropin Releasing Hormone Agonists
GYN	Gynecology
HCG	Human chorionic gonadotropin
HIPAA	Health Insurance Portability and Accounting Act of 1996
HMB	Heavy menstrual bleeding
HMOs	Health maintenance organizations
HPV	Human papilloma virus
HRT	Hormone replacement therapy
HSV	Herpes Simplex Virus
HTN	Hypertension
IC	Interstitial Cystitis

IUPC	Intrauterine pressure catheter
JC	Joint Commission
LAVH	Laparoscopic assisted vaginal hysterectomy
LMP	Last menstrual period
LSH	Laparoscopic supracervical hysterectomy
MCA	Middle cerebral artery
MFM	Maternal fetal medicine specialist
MOC	Maintenance of Certification
MRI	Magnetic resonance imaging
NSAIDs	Nonsteroidal anti-inflammatory drugs
OAB	Overactive bladder
OB	Obstetrics
OCPs	Oral contraceptive pills
P	Parity
PACU	Post anesthesia care unit
PALM-COEIN	PALM-COEIN system for AUB
PAR	Post anesthesia recovery room
PCOS	Polycystic ovarian syndrome
PID	Pelvic inflammatory disease
PMP	Postmenopausal
PPTL	Postpartum tubal ligation
PPROM	Preterm prolonged rupture of membranes
PROM	Prolonged rupture of membranes
POD	Postoperative day
REI	Reproductive endocrinology infertility
RR	Recovery room
SCIP	Surgical Care Improvement Project
SIL	Squamous intraepithelial lesion
SOB	Shortness of breath
S/P	Status post
SPVT	Septic pelvic vein thrombosis
SROM	Spontaneous rupture of membranes
STD	Sexually transmitted disease
SUI	Stress urinary incontinence
TAH	Total abdominal hysterectomy
TOLAC	Trial of labor after cesarean delivery
TLH	Total laparoscopic hysterectomy
TVH	Transvaginal or total vaginal hysterectomy
UI	Urinary incontinence
U/S	Ultrasound
UTI	Urinary tract infection
VBAC	Vaginal birth after cesarean section
VH	Vaginal hysterectomy
VIN	Vulvar intraepithelial neoplasia
V/Q	Ventilation-perfusion scan

Appendix C

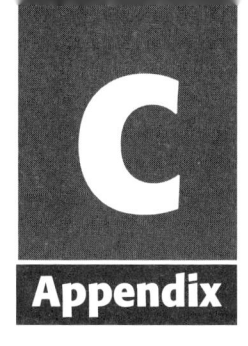

Addresses

American Board of Obstetrics and Gynecology, Inc.
2915 Vine Street, Suite 300
Dallas, TX 75204-1069
Phone: (214) 871-1619
Fax: (214) 871-1943
e-mail: info@abog.org
http://www.abog.org

American College of Obstetricians and Gynecologists
409 12th Street, S.W., P.O. Box 96920
Washington, DC 20090-6920
Phone: (202) 638-5577
1-800-673-8444
Fax: (202) 484-5107
e-mail: use initial of first name followed by up to seven characters of the last name followed by @acog.com
http://www.acog.org

For publications: ACOG Distribution Center, 1-800-762-2264 or http://www.acog.org

America's OB/GYN Board Review Course
   53 Gary Hill Drive, Suite 10
   East Flat Rock, NC 28726
   Phone: 1-877-ABC-OBGYN (1-877-222-6249)
   FAX: (828) 698-5510
   e-mail: info@americasboardreview.com
   http://www.americasboardreview.com

Author of This Book
   A. Krishna Das, MD, FACOG
   622 Sabine Drive
   Hendersonville, NC 28739
   Cellular phone: (828) 606-6956
   Fax: (828) 687-1814
   e-mail: krisdas@americasboardreview.com
   or
   krisdas@morrisbb.net

Appendix D

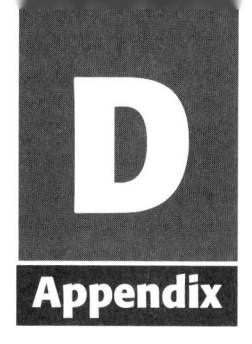

Custom Case List

The most influential factor for passing your test is your case list. Henceforth, it is imperative that you strategically construct it to put your best foot forward. Remember, your examiner sees your case list before he even shakes your hand; therefore, his first impression of you is based entirely on your case list.

Your priority is to construct the best case list possible. It is absolutely imperative that you select the case list software that will best help you meet your goals. You have two options: you can either purchase pre-existing case list software or you can create your own. Let's review the pros and cons of each.

ABOG Software

ABOG has software that you may obtain by simply ordering online at abog.org. Candidates erroneously assume that it is mandatory to use the ABOG software. This is simply NOT true. You may use ANY format, as long as it exactly duplicates the ABOG case list forms.

In my opinion, the ABOG software is the least preferable option. ACOG was the first to author the software in the early 1990s and then relinquished it over to ABOG in the early 2000s. As with any project, each revision improves on the last; however, it still continues to have many limitations.

The ABOG program is not very user friendly. You have little control of the order of cases and editing within each case. The ABOG software will not let you easily make logical word breaks in columns or pages, nor can you align your flow of thought from one column to the next. Finally, the ABOG software doesn't track statistics accurately for your summary sheets.

The overall impression is that this software is inferior compared to the other options available. An ABOG-generated case list does not present as well and is not optimal in strategic construction. Consistently, a chief regret of past candidates is that they used the ABOG software. Unfortunately, you have not reviewed many case lists, if any, and just have to trust me on this. All I can say is after having reviewed hundreds, perhaps thousands, of case lists over more than 25 years, a well-constructed case list is truly OUTSTANDING compared to the majority that settle for mainstream.

At the beginning of your case list collection, you're at a loss as to where to begin. I would start with the ABOG software, because it's turnkey. However, once you have the basics and begin to experience frustration with the software's limitations, I would bail. If you are entering your cases in a timely fashion (eg. every 1-2 weeks), you will quickly recognize the format and information required for your case collection. You can then decide whether you'd like to continue to use the ABOG software, switch to a different software program or create a custom case list. You should be making this decision to unload the unwanted ballast by the spring.

So, if not the ABOG program, then what? You have two remaining options. Purchase a different commercial software or create your own. Let's review the pros and cons of each.

Commercial Software

There are a number of commercial software products available. ABOG will bias you against others, as even in their application acceptance letter it states that "commercially available programs do no print an acceptable case list". My experience has been that most commercial software is better than the ABOG software. However, like any software designed by someone else, you are subject to their rules, biases and formatting. Plus, your case list will look like all the others that have used the same software. So ironically, you're right back to the problem of blending in with the rest of the crowd.

Additionally, commercial products cost more when compared to the ABOG software. Furthermore, you must be careful that the software is up-to-date and reflects the latest ABOG changes. Remember, your case list format must exactly reproduce that required by ABOG. Finally, if their technical support is unsatisfactory, this can leave you in a pickle, especially if the August 1st due date is looming overhead.

Customized Case List

Your final option is to create your own case list program. This is initially the most time consuming, but also assures your case list will conform entirely to *your* standard. NO ONE will have a case list that looks like yours. You WILL stand out.

The best case list I have EVER seen was from a candidate nearing retirement! I had two questions for him: 1) "Why on earth are you taking the test now?" and 2) "HOW did/could you construct such a beautiful case list?".

His response to my first question was that this was something he wanted to do for himself before he died. Many years ago, neither the emphasis on, nor the mandate for, board certification existed as it does now. He never needed board certification to practice, but he prided himself on always keeping up to date. This was his last validation of a successful career… and something he wanted to quietly achieve for himself.

His response to my second question was quite simple. His *high school* son created the case list! His son was entering the data in the then ACOG software. It had so many glitches, he, *on his own*, created the custom software!

Most of you are of the same generation as his son (born since the 1980s), so you can easily do the same. I was lecturing at a review course on this topic and showed the audience an example of the above case list. An inspired candidate approached me the NEXT day with a draft of her attempt. It was good, but I felt it could be better. To make a long story short, it only took her three consecutive evenings (after having sat through 10 hours of lectures) to program a stellar case list. I have had this same story repeated time after time. Literally, designing the template only takes a few hours. In addition, your custom template will probably save you many hours later, since editing your Word or Excel document is a lot easier than changing formatting or entries on someone else's case list software. Here's how to create your very own.

Paradigm Shift

Recall that in Chapter 5, The Case List and also in Chapter 9, Image Enhancement, we discussed the necessity to step out of your shoes and into the examiner's. You need to undergo a paradigm shift and look at your case list as if you were the examiner.

Pick up your own or anybody else's case list. What cases would you ask about? *Why* would you ask about those cases? Chances are, because it was an interesting or unusual topic or perhaps because of the complication that ensued. Whatever the reason, you can use this to your advantage simply by making that word(s) stand out and catch your eye. You can use **bold**, CAPITALIZE, underline, or *italicize* that key word. How about even highlighting or shading the whole column? Physically changing the keyword or phrase will involuntarily pull the eye to that word. GOTCHA! Now the examiner may acknowledge that yes indeed, this is something he would like to ask about. And you are so ready for him, because you set the bait.

Remember, many of your examiners are over forty and wear bifocals. ABOG mandates that the size of the print be 10-point. How about carrying that a step further? Your software should give you the freedom to design and organize to your choosing. You can insert horizontal tracking lines to follow the flow within and between columns. Consider leaving a space between patients. Place vertical tracking lines to demarcate columns. A most elegant organizational tool is bullets. Will your software allow you to insert them?

Finally, make sure your software allows you ease in editing. You shouldn't have to struggle and redo the whole page just to add or delete words. Also, you must be able to control where your word is hyphenated within a column. An absolute no-no is to carry a case over to the next page.

If I've convinced you, at least philosophically, to consider customizing your case list, the next step is logistics. Believe it or not, this is the easy and rewarding part.

Software

Obviously there are a number of software products on the market. You should choose the one with which you are the most comfortable, as well as that which is the most capable of producing the desired product. The most common is Microsoft Word or Microsoft Excel.

My preference for a customized case list is Microsoft Word. Although it is primarily utilized for entering and editing straight text, it has significant formatting muscle that can help make your case list outstanding. Below, you will read what pertinent heading information and categories must be included in each section of the case list. Since each section of the case list is a bit different, you will need three different formatted documents: one for each of the Obstetrics, Gynecology and Office Practice cases. Don't fret! Once you get one of them figured out, the other case list sections are easily created.

Appendix D • Custom Case List

The first step in your Word document is to create a header to be inserted at the top of each page. Mandatory information to be included in the header is: the page number, your name, case list number and whether these are post residency, fellowship or senior residency cases. (See Example 1) You can also include in the header the column titles for that specific section. (See Example 2) For example, on your Office Practice case list, you would include everything from Patient number to the number of patient visits.

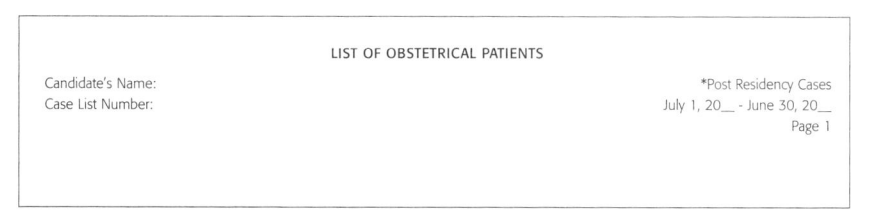

	LIST OF OBSTETRICAL PATIENTS	
Candidate's Name: Case List Number:		*Post Residency Cases July 1, 20__ - June 30, 20__ Page 1

Example 1

						LIST OF OBSTETRICAL PATIENTS							
Candidate's Name: Case List Number:												*Post Residency Cases July 1, 20__ - June 30, 20__ Page 1	
Case #	Hosp #	Pate #	Age	Grav	Para	Complications			Days in Hosp	Newborn			
						Antepartum	Delivery or Postpartum	Operative Procedure and/or Treatments		Perinatal Death	Wgt Gms	Apgars 1/5 Mins	Days in Hosp

Example 2

Your two biggest challenges will be to choose an acceptable font that can be easily read, and also make your margins small enough to fit everything. Now you need to decide on left or center alignments, as well as top and bottom alignments for each column heading. That's it! Since this is now in your Word header, it will automatically appear on every page of your case list.

The second part of your Word document will be the actual body of the document. Now create a table that lines up exactly with the column headings that you just created in your header. If your header has 15 columns, then so will your main content in the body of the document. Once that is done, you are ready to start entering data. (See Example 3)

LIST OF OBSTETRICAL PATIENTS

Candidate's Name:
Case List Number:

*Post Residency Cases
July 1, 20__ - June 30, 20__
Page 1

Case #	Hosp #	Patea #	Age	Grava	Para	Complications			Days in Hosp	Newborn		
						Antepartum	Delivery or Postpartum	Operative Procedure and/or Treatments		Perinatal Death	Wgt Gms	Apgars 1/5 Mins	Days in Hosp

Obstetrical Categories _____

Example 3

I would recommend trying out just 3 or 4 cases to see how it will look, before diving into entering your data. Basically, each case is a new row in your table. By entering a few cases, you will then be able to experiment with other types of formatting options. Should you use bullets? What do you want them to look like? Where do you want to use them? Which font looks better? Make sure your font is not the same as ABOG's or the other commercial products. I suggest Arial font. How can you best clarify your patient management?

Furthermore, you can insert a new row for each of your categories. A snazzy look is to then merge the cells in that row so it can fit all the way across. To make a new area stand out even more, you can use light colored shading in that new row, or perhaps bold your chosen font for the category headings. (See Example 4). You will have to see what is pleasing to your eye, although I would recommend staying on the conservative side when it comes to shading.

You can apply the same methods to Excel. The advantage is that the Excel worksheet is already a table. However, I feel the formatting options for text is not as viable as with Word.

Regardless of which program you decide to use to create your case list, have fun with it and let the creative juices flow! Just remember to stay within the minimal guidelines laid out by ABOG. Finally, remember to back up your case list frequently! If your computer dies during your year of case collection, you will be sorry!

Appendix D • Custom Case List

Candidate's Name:
Caselist Number: 123456

Post Residency Cases
July 1, 20___ - June 30, 20___
Page 1

LIST OF OBSTETRICAL PATIENTS

Hosp #	Pat age	G R a v	P A R A	G P A	GEST AGE	COMPLICATIONS			OPERATIVE PROCEDURES AND/OR TREATMENT	DAYS IN HOSP	NEWBORN			
						ANTEPARTUM	DELIVERY OR POSTPARTUM				PERI-NATAL DEATH	WGT gms	APGAR 1/5 MIN	DAYS IN HOSP

Example 4

Setting Up Your Own Database

Creating your database or template is the biggest challenge. Once it is set, making the case list is simply a matter of data entry. Your database must comply exactly with the ABOG specifications. Check the ABOG website for the most up-to-date forms. Your initial packet from ABOG includes these specifications, as well as sample pages for the three sections (Examples 5, 6, and 7), the summary sheet (Examples 8, 9, and 10) and the affidavit sheet (see below).

Each page of the case list has a heading (List of Obstetric Patients, List of Gynecologic Patients or List of Office Practice Patients), page number, your name, case list number and whether they are post residency, fellowship or senior residency cases. Each section (Obstetrics, Gynecology, or Office) has specific columns to list each case. Each respective section (Ob, Gyn, or Office) should begin with page number 1 and be numbered consecutively thereafter. Furthermore, each patient should be numbered consecutively so every patient has a unique number, as well. Refer to Chapter 5 for a list of categories for each section. If you do not have a patient in one of the categories, still list the category heading, but specify "None" on the form.

AFFIDAVIT SHEET FOR EACH SITE

Candidate's Name: _____
Hospital: _____
Hospital Address: _____
             Street   City, State   Zip Code

ATTEST: The patients listed on pages _____ through _____ include ALL hospitalized patients discharged or transferred from the care of DOCTOR _____ at this hospital (site) from _____
to _____
                     (Date)

Signature and Title of Hospital (site) Official
(e.g., Medical Record Administrator or Other): _____
                     (Signature)

                     (Title)

Signature of the Candidate: _____

The American Board of Obstetrics and Gynecology reserves the right to audit the accuracy of this list.

Obstetrical Case List Forms

☐ Post Residency Cases   ☐ Senior Residency Cases   ☐ Fellowship Cases

#	HOSP #	PAT #	AGE	GRAV	PARA	Gest Age	COMPLICATIONS		Operative Procedures And/or Treatment	Days In Hosp. (Not Dates)	NEWBORN			
							Antepartum	Delivery or Postpartum			Perinatal Death	Wgt	APGAR 1 & 5 Minutes	Days In Hosp. (Not Dates)

I. Number of Uncomplicated Spontaneous Deliveries _____
II. Obstetrical Categories (1-31) _____
III. Total number of <u>ultrasound</u> and <u>Color Doppler examinations</u> performed by you upon hospitalized obstetrical patients _____
IV. Total number of:
    A. APGAR scores 5 or less _____
    B. Infants < 2500 gms _____
    C. Perinatal Deaths _____

* Patients' names, initials, and hospital names must not be used. Also, patients who are over 89 years of age must not have their age listed.

\# refers to a sequential ordering which is assigned by the computer for ALL patients from all hospitals, i.e., 1-xxx.

Hospital # refers to the sequential ordering of hospitals being reported from, i.e.,   Hospital A = First hospital from which patients are being reported; Hospital B = Second hospital from which patients are being reported.

Hospital C = Third hospital from which patients are being reported.

Patient # refers to a sequential ordering of patients reported from a given hospital, i.e., Hospital A, patients 1-x; Hospital B, patients 1-xx.

Example 5

Pass Your Oral OB/GYN Board Exam!

Gynecological Case List Forms

LIST OF GYNECOLOGICAL PATIENTS*	☐ Post Residency Cases	☐ Senior Residency Cases	☐ Fellowship Cases

H O S P #	P A T #	A G E	G R A V	P A R A	DIAGNOSIS PREOPERATIVE OR ADMISSION	TREATMENT	SURGICAL PATHOLOGY DIAGNOSIS (Uterine Wt. in gms.)	COMPLICATIONS (Include blood transfusions)	Days In Hosp. (Not Dates)

i. Gynecological Categories (1-29)
ii. Total number of <u>ultrasound</u> and <u>Color Doppler Examinations</u> performed by you upon hospitalized gynecological patients _____

* Patients' names, initials, and hospital names must not be used. Also, patients who are over 89 years of age must not have their age listed.

\# refers to a sequential ordering which is assigned by the computer for ALL patients from all hospitals, i.e., 1-xxx.

Hospital # refers to the sequential ordering of hospitals being reported from, i.e., Hospital A = First hospital from which patients are being reported;
Hospital B = Second hospital from which patients are being reported;
Hospital C = Third hospital from which patients are being reported.

Patient # refers to a sequential ordering of patients reported from a given hospital, i.e., Hospital A, patients 1-x; Hospital B, patients 1-xx.

Example 6

Appendix D • Custom Case List

Office Practice Case List Forms

LIST OF OFFICE PRACTICE PATIENTS*

#	AGE	GRAV	PARA	PROBLEM	DIAGNOSTIC PROCEDURES	TREATMENT	RESULTS	No. of Visits

I. Office Practice Categories (1–40)
II. Total Number of <u>Ultrasound</u> and <u>Color Doppler Examinations</u> in:
   A. Obstetrical patients _____
   B. Gynecological patients _____
   C. Other areas such as abdominal, thoracic, pediatric, etc. _____

* Patient's names, initials and hospital names must not be used. Also, patients who are over 89 years of age must not have their age listed.

\# refers to a sequential ordering which is assigned by the computer for ALL patients from all hospitals, i.e., 1-xxx.

The American Board of Obstetrics and Gynecology offers a case list collection and reporting software program for the oral examination (available on-line or email caselists@abog.org or phone 214 871-1619)

Example 7

Pass Your Oral OB/GYN Board Exam!

Candidate's Name _____   Case List ID # _____   Date Range of Case List _____

SUMMARY SHEET/ALL HOSPITALS AND AMBULATORY SURGICAL SITES COMBINED

A. GYNECOLOGIC CATEGORIES	Total Cases	Total Applied	A. GYNECOLOGIC CATEGORIES	Total Cases	Total Applied
Abdominal Hysterectomy			Postoperative Wound Complications		
Laparotomy (Other than Tubal Sterilization)			Postoperative Thrombophlebitis and/or Embolism		
Vaginal Hysterectomy (Including Laparoscopically Assisted)			Postoperative Fever for Greater than 48 hours		
			Rectovaginal or Urinary Tract Fistula		
Diagnostic Laparoscopy			Culposcopy		
Operative Laparoscopy (Other than Tubal Sterilization)			TOTAL CASES		
Operative Hysteroscopy					
Uterine Myomas			B. NUMBER OF HOSPITAL STAYS > 7 DAYS		
Defects in Pelvic Floor					
Endometriosis			C. GYNECOLOGIC ULTRASOUNDS & DOPPLER EXAMINATIONS		
Tubal Sterilization					
Invasive Carcinoma					
Carcinoma in situ					
Infertility Evaluation					
Infertility Treatment					
Urinary Incontinence					
Urinary Incontinence (Surgical Treatment)					
Ectopic Pregnancy					
Abdominal Hysterectomy					
Pelvic Pain					
Congenital Abnormalities of the Reproductive Tract					
Pelvic Inflammatory Disease					
Adnexal Problems excluding Ectopic Pregnancy and Pelvic Inflammatory Disease					
Abnormal Uterine Bleeding					
Vulvar Masses					
Vulvar Ulcers					
Adenomyosis					

Example 8

Appendix D • Custom Case List

Candidate's Name _____ Case List ID # _____ Date Range of Case List _____

SUMMARY SHEET/ALL HOSPITALS AND AMBULATORY SURGICAL SITES COMBINED

A. OBSTETRIC CATEGORIES	Total Cases	Total Applied	A. OBSTETRIC CATEGORIES	Total Cases	Total Applied
Breech and Other Fetal Malpresentations			Pregnancies Complicated by Human Immunodeficiency Virus Infection (HIV)		
Intrapartum Infection (Amnionitis)			Primary Cesarean Delivery		
Puerperal Infection			Repeat Cesarean Delivery		
Third Trimester Bleeding			Inductions and/or Augmentations of Labor		
Multifetal Pregnancy			Puerpal Hemorrhage		
Cesarean Pregnancy			Readmission for Maternal Complication Up to 6 Weeks Postpartum		
Premature Rupture of Fetal Membranes at Term			TOTAL CASES		
Preterm Premature Rupture of Membranes			B. TOTAL UNCOMPLICATED SPONTANEOUS DELIVERIES		
Preterm Delivery					
Hypertensive Disorders of Pregnancy (Chronic hypertension, preeclampsia, eclampsia)			C. OBSTETRIC ULTRASOUNDS & DOPPLER EXAMINATIONS		
Second Trimester Spontaneous Abortion			D. NUMBER OF OTHER OBSTETRICAL CONSIDERATIONS		
Cardiovascular and/or Pulmonary Diseases Complicating Pregnancy			1. Apgar Scores 5 or less		
Renal Diseases and/or Neurological Diseases Complicating Pregnancy			2. Infants < 2500 gms		
Hematological Disease and/or Endocrine Diseases Complicating Pregnancy			3. Perinatal deaths		
Infections Complicating Pregnancy					
Postterm Pregnancy					
Abnormal Fetal Growth					
Vaginal Birth After Cesarean Delivery					
Any Maternal Complication which Delayed Maternal Hospital Discharge by 48 or More Hours					
Any Neonatal Complication which Delayed Neonatal Hospital Discharge by 48 or More Hours					
Pregnancies Complicated by Fetal Anomalies					

Example 9

Candidate's Name _____ Case List ID # _____ Date Range of Case List _____

SUMMARY SHEET/ALL HOSPITALS AND AMBULATORY SURGICAL SITES COMBINED

A. OFFICE PRACTICE CATEGORIES	Total Cases	Total Applied	A. OFFICE PRACTICE CATEGORIES	Total Cases	Total Applied
Preventive Care and Health Maintenance			Spousal Abuse		
Counseling for Smoking Cessation and Treatment of Obesity			Dysmenorrhea		
Counseling for Sexual Dysfunction			Premenstrual Syndrome		
Contraception			Benign Pelvic Masses		
Psychosomatic Problems			Vaginal Ultrasonography		
Genetic Counseling			Back Pain		
Primary or Secondary Amenorrhea			Respiratory Tract Diseases		
Hirsutism			Gastrointestinal Diseases		
Irfertility			Cardiovascular Diseases		
Hyperprolactinemia			Endocrine Diseases (Diabetes Mellitus, Thyroid or Adrenal Disease)		
Endometriosis			Hypertension		
Menopausal Care			Diagnosis and Management of Hypercholesterolemia and Dyslipidemias		
Office Surgery			Recognition and Counseling for Substance Abuse (Alcohol, Narcotics, etc.)		
Abnormal Uterine Bleeding			Depression		
Abnormal Cervical Cytology			Geriatrics		
Pelvic Pain					
Vaginal Discharge					
Vulvar Disease					
Breast Diseases					
Urinary Incontinence and Pelvic Floor Defects					
Urinary Tract Infections					
Sexually Transmitted Diseases					
Preconceptional Counseling					
Immunizations					
Pediatric Gynecology					
Sexual Assault					

Example 10

Setting Up Your Obstetric Database

The obstetric list is subcategorized into Number of Uncomplicated Spontaneous Deliveries, Obstetrical Categories, Total Number of Ultrasound and Color Doppler Examinations Performed by You Upon Hospitalized Obstetrical Patients, and Total number of APGAR scores of 5 or less, Infants < 2500 grams, and Perinatal Deaths. You can make the categories stand out by shadowing the title (Example 11). The column headings are as follows:

Patient's case list number	Operative procedures and/or treatment
Patient's hospital number	Patient's number of days in the hospital
Age	Newborn perinatal death
Gravida	Newborn weight
Parity	Apgars at 1 and 5 minutes
Gestational age	Newborn days in hospital
Complications of antepartum	
Complications of delivery or postpartum	

The most challenging part of designing your obstetric list is to fit all the columns on one page. As more information is entered, the print becomes smaller and more difficult to read. Try the following tricks to make this section look its best:

1. Be sure to use the landscape orientation on your document.
2. Make the left and right margins as wide as possible and narrow the non-complication columns.
3. Use a large, easy-on-the-eye font. (ABOG mandates 10 point.) Experiment with different fonts until you find one you like.
3. Use a large, easy-on-the-eye font. (ABOG mandates 10 point.) Experiment with different fonts until you find one you like.
4. List the required information vertically rather than horizontally within a column to save space and, more importantly, to align flow of thought between columns. Using formatting bullets will help you with vertical listing. Draw a horizontal line between cases. Limit each page to six or so cases; a longer list results in eye strain and overwhelms the reader with too much data.

LIST OF OBSTETRIC PATIENTS

Candidate's name _____   July 1, ____ —June 30, ____   Page 1

Initials & Hosp. No.	Age	Gravida	Para	Gest. Age	Antepartum	Complications Delivery or Postpartum	Opertive Procedures and/or Treatment	Days in Hosp.	Newborn Complications	Wgt. (gm)	Apgar 1 & 5 Minutes	Days in Hosp.
A. Antepartum Admissions												
B. Obstetric Deliveries												
C. Other Obstetric Considerations												
D. Postpartum Readmissions												
E. Patients Transfused												
Total Normal, Uncomplicated Obstetric Patients												
Total Number of Ultrasound and Doppler Examinations on Hospitalized Obstetric Patients												

Example 11

Setting Up Your Gynecologic Database

The gynecologic case list is subcategorized into the categories listed on the summary sheet. The column headings are as follows:

    Patient's case list number   Diagnosis (preoperative or admission)
    Patient's hospital number   Treatment
    Patient's number   Surgical pathology diagnosis
    Age   Complications
    Gravida   Number of days hospitalized
    Parity

   Because there are fewer columns than with the obstetric case list, it is easier to fit all data on one page. However, the same recommendations to enhance readability apply. Remember to start over on the page count and the patient numbering. Do not forget to include size (cm) for ovarian cysts, weight (grams) for uterine pathology and blood transfusions for complications. Examples 12 and 13 are ideal in presentation and content. Notice the proper use of bullets, cases per page, and abbreviations.

Setting Up Your Office Practice Database

The office practice case list has 37 categories to choose from (see Chapter 5). You may list only 40 patients and no more than 2 patients per category. List all the categories but annotate "None observed" when appropriate. The ABOG program does not list the category if there are no representative patients. You are prone to then forget about these categories (out of sight, out of mind), yet you will still be accountable for all 37 categories. Because there are fewer columns, it is very easy to include all the information on one page. Remember to reset both the page number and the patient numbering. Example 14 is an excellent representation of a cleanly designed list.

   The column headings are as follows:

    Patient's number   Problem
    Age   Diagnostic procedures
    Gravida   Treatment
    Parity   Results
    Number of patient visits

LIST OF GYNECOLOGIC PATIENTS

1 July - 30 June

Candidate's Name: __John Q. Doe__

List ALL gynecology patients in each hospital or clinical site in the following order:
I. Hospitalized patients: A. Major operative procedures, B. Minor operative procedures, C. Nonsurgical admissions, D. Total number of ultrasound and Doppler examinations performed by you upon hospitalized gynecologic patients.
II. Ambulatory or Short-stay surgery gynecology patients.

#	Initials & Hosp. No.	Age	Gravida	Para	Diagnosis Preoperative or Admission (include size of ovarian cysts)	Treatment	Surgical Pathology Diagnosis (uterine wt. in gms.)	Complications (include blood transfusions)	Days in Hosp.
	TM 250906	33	0	0	• Stage IV endometriosis • Failure to control pain with 3 prior laparoscopies and medical management	• TAH/BSO • Extensive lysis of adhesions	Uterus - 121gm • Endometriosis • Adenomyosis Cervix - benign	• Vaginal cuff abscess	4
B. Minor Operative Procedures									
	CB 048942	50	2	2	• Postoperative vaginal cuff abscess	• Colpotomy, drainage and culture • Intravenous antibiotics	• Mixed anaerobes	• None	2
C. Nonsurgical Admissions									
		50	2	2	• Anemia, ascites, alcoholism • Consulted for presumed HMB	• Pad count • Endometrial biopsy • Consulted for presumed HMB	• Proliferative endometrium	• None	12
	DR 127386	32	4	3	• Ectopic pregnancy treated with methotrexate 4 days prior to admission • Worsening pain	• Close observation • Serial blood counts • Serial quantitative HCG	• N/A	• None	1

Example 12

Appendix D • Custom Case List

LIST OF GYNECOLOGIC PATIENTS

1 July - 30 June

Candidate's Name: _____ Hospital Name: _____

#	Initials & Hosp. No.	Age	Gravida	Para	Diagnosis Preoperative or Admission (include size of ovarian cysts)	Treatment	Surgical Pathology Diagnosis (uterine wt. in gms.)	Complications (include blood transfusions)	Days in Hosp.
1	D.H. 601512	44	4	4	• HMB • Right adnexal mass: 6 × 7 cm	• TAH—BSO	Uterus - 184gm • Adenomyosis R ovary - • Papillary serous cystadenoma L ovary - benign	None	2
B. Other Laparotomies									
2	T.G. 361206	29	3	1	• Acute abdomen • Rule out ruptured ectopic pregnancy	• Laparotomy • Right salpingectomy	• Ectopic tubal gestation • Hematosalpinx • Hemoperitoneum	Anemia	2
3	J.F. 904281	27	4	1	• Rule out ectopic pregnancy	• Diagnostic laparoscopy • Laparotomy • Right cornual pregnancy	• Right tubal pregnancy	Anemia	2
4	J.E. 675902	37	6	3	• Missed Ab • Rule out ectopic pregnancy	• Suction D&C • Diagnostic laparoscopy • Laparotomy • Right salpingectomy	• Right tubal pregnancy	None	2

Example 13

LIST OF OUTPATIENTS

Barbara Angelika Dill, M.D.

July 1, 1996–June 30, 1997

#	Initials	Age	Gravida	Para	Problem	Diagnostic Procedures	Treatment	Results	No. of Visits
I. Patient List									
Preoperative Care & Health Maintenance									
153	RA	35	3	2	Annual exam Polycystic ovary disease	Pap, baseline mammogram, lipid profile, 2h glucose test	Dietary modification	Elevated cholesterol Glucose normal	2
154	AG	73	0	0	Annual exam Breast cancer × 1 yr on tamoxifen Vaginal pruritus	Pap Endometrial biopsy: atrophic	Topical estrogen (discussed with breast surgeon and oncologist)	Resolution	3
Obesity									
None observed									
Sexual Dysfunction									
155	ME	50	2	4	Decreased libido on HRT	None	Testosterone added to HRT	Improvement	6
Contraceptive Complications									
156	BB	31	0	0	Amenorrhea on oral contraceptives	Pregnancy test: negative	Changed strength from 20 mg to 30 mg	Regular menses	2
157	VM	63	5	5	Postmenopausal bleeding IUD perforating through cervix	IUD culture: actinomycoses Endometrial biopsy: atrophic	IUD removal PCN G 500 qd × 4 wk	No recurrence	6
Psychomatic Problems									
None observed									

Example 14

Appendix D • Custom Case List

If you have more specific questions on how to create a custom case list, contact me (See Appendix C for contact information) and I can connect you with some clever consultants who can assist you.

In conclusion, you have three software options to enter your data: ABOG, another commercial product or design your own. Although all meet the ABOG criteria, the customized software is the most likely to result in a polished product that stands out from the rest. Given that half of the exam is based on the case list and your case list makes the first impression, seize the opportunity to use this to your complete advantage.

Appendix E

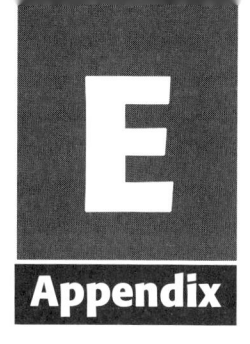

Recommendations for Subspecialty Fellows

The pressing issue on most subspecialty fellows' minds is *when* to take their general boards exam. One thing for certain, you cannot sit for your subspecialty oral boards until you pass your general oral board exam. You will be horrified to acknowledge how much you have forgotten about your non-subspecialty areas. For this reason, I recommend you take your general board exam as soon as possible.

Effective in 2013, you can sit for your exam anytime during your fellowship. Of course, not all fellowship directors are in open support of this and some may discourage you from taking it until your third research year. You will forget so quickly those off-specialty topics. The longer you wait, the worse the recall. If you're no longer practicing general OB/GYN, you peaked in your chief residency year. Back then, it was inconceivable that you could ever forget how to deliver a baby or perform a hysterectomy, since you could practically do it in your sleep. However, it's true - if you don't use it, you'll lose it. You need to persuade your fellowship director that it's to the program's advantage for you to take the exam as soon as possible, in order to enhance your chances of passing and also to assure your program's excellent reputation.

I strongly recommend you apply for your basic oral exam the first year of your fellowship. Specifically, you took your primary written board exam at the end of June of your chief residency year and you started your fellowship on July 1. You won't even get your written exam results until September 1, so you will need to apply for the accelerated or fast track.

This means you need to start collecting cases day one of the first year of your fellowship. However, remember the earliest you can then sit for your oral boards won't be until the fall of your second year of your fellowship.

Since 2006, every page of your case list is stamped "fellow". So it's like a billboard with flashing lights announcing your title. Heck, it's pretty obvious upon a mere glance of your case list by the type of cases anyway...that is, if one looks at the entire list. Unfortunately though, this is not the case, as each examiner receives only his portion. So if you're an Oncologist, the only clue to your OB examiner is the "fellow" box checked at the top, but he doesn't know if you're Oncology, REI, FPM, MIS, etc.

As a fellow or subspecialist in your chief year, you are allowed to submit a case list of 20 hospitalized or surgical patients in your non-subspecialty. I so hope you proactive folk are reading this now to remind you to save that doggone chief residency log for your non-specialty case list. It is a pathetic sight to witness a fellow discovering this after the fact. Choose bread and butter cases, not esoteric ones. Also, go on the heavy side of content, because this is a legal cheat sheet. You're going to need all the help you can get. The *Bulletin* is inconsistent, but sometimes you are limited to exactly 20 cases and sometimes not. If not, then go beyond 20 to add depth and breadth, plus this will force you to know beyond those 20 patients. If possible, sign up to cover the resident clinic or take ED or L&D call. This will add to your list, but more importantly, help to keep your fingers nimble. The candidate who can readily tap into their everyday clinical practice during the exam is at an advantage. Even though your case list may be limited, you will still be examined in all three areas: obstetrics, gynecology, and office practice.

The office practice case list consists only of patients from your current practice. So your office list is usually another give-away of your specialty. For example, if you're an MFM, all of your patients are pregnant or postpartum; likewise, if you're an oncologist, all of your patients have, or had, cancer. However, the purpose of the office list is general gynecology. So the examiner will wiggle her nose and poof! make the cancer and pregnancy go away. While you're constructing your list and preparing your defense, keep this in mind. For example, under the "Endocrine Diseases eg. Diabetes Mellitus" category, recognize that the focus for the gestational diabetic patient you listed will be on screening and diagnosis in a non-pregnant state or her risk for developing diabetes later in life.

Most importantly, keep in mind that you are sitting for the *general* boards, not your subspecialty boards. You are expected to have the same knowledge base in *all three* areas as any other candidate.

Appendix D • Recommendations for Subspecialty Fellows

Undoubtedly your clinical acumen in your subspecialty will be above and beyond what is expected for the general boards. But the goal is not to verify your expertise in your subspecialty; your time will come when you sit for your subspecialty boards. So don't waste a lot of time in constructing your specialty cases. They will go on ad nauseam and if you've seen one, you've seen them all. Keep the detail to a minimum.

Therefore, starting right now, spend no further time on studying your subspecialty. Your energy should be devoted to refreshing your grasp of the basics in the other areas you used to know. Prioritize studying the topics you know are going to be on the test. The list is as follows:

1. "Know Cold" topics - Chapter 8 Table 1
2. "Hot" topics - Chapter 8 Table 2
3. "Case of the Day" - Chapter 7 Tables 1, 2, 3

Limiting your studying to these topics alone will cover at least 80% of your exam.

While studying, keep in mind you need to know only the basics to pass the question. You have become accustomed to knowing even the most trivial minutiae and ground-breaking research in your subspecialty. Refrain from trying to achieve the same depth in the general topics. Not only will you waste precious time, but you do not get extra credit for going beyond the required threshold.

A board review course is essential. A good course should give you 90% of all you need to know for your off-specialty topics. It will help to hold back the reins on going above and beyond. Additionally, it will reintroduce your specialty from the generalist's perspective. You've lost this view, as you're accustomed to the generalist neatly packaging up the patient and depositing her on your doorstep. You need to recapture all that happens prior to you receiving her.

The general exam is quite humbling. You are respected and recognized for your expertise in your subspecialty. You know a lot about one area; now you need to know a little about everything again. It is amazing how much you have forgotten about the other areas.

There are only two reasons that a fellow fails his general oral board exam. The first is a pompous, "know-it-all" attitude. This fellow cannot resist belittling the examiner and debating with him at the same or higher level on the fellow's subspecialty topic. The second reason is failure to demonstrate a minimal knowledge base in non-subspecialty topics.

In conclusion, remember that you are taking your general boards. You need to demonstrate the same knowledge base in all three areas as any other candidate. No extra credit is given for going above and beyond the mandatory threshold. But you will certainly fail if you do not know your basics. Do not be arrogant and demeaning. Swallow your pride and join the ranks with the generalists.

Appendix F

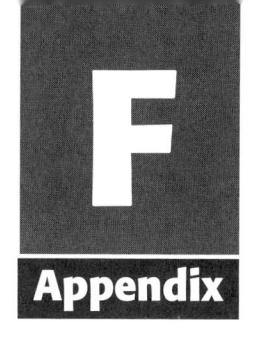

Recommendations for Military Personnel

The primary reason for seeking board certification is probably the same for civilian and military physicians. Some incentives, however, are unique to the military.

If you are board-certified, you receive a monthly bonus stipend. Furthermore, board certification influences your assignment of duty position and station. You are more likely to be assigned to a sought-after teaching facility if you are board-certified. Certainly board certification makes you marketable if you decide to leave the military.

Historically, military personnel enjoy an excellent track record. Statistically as a group, you have a nearly 100% pass rate. Are you better trained? I doubt it, since most of you were trained in civilian residencies. The explanation probably lies in the unique differences and challenges of practicing Ob/Gyn in the military.

It usually becomes obvious when you are defending your case list that you lack the support of both Ob/Gyn and other colleagues because of the omnipresent physician shortage in the military. Ancillary resources are restricted because of geographical limitations and shortages. Your patient population is different. Deployments, missions, and nontraditional job duties often influence timing and urgency for evaluation, management, and follow-up. Thus, you must be more creative, broad-based, resourceful, and independent than your civilian colleagues. Examiners love it!

The examiner can tell instantly that you are in the military from the name of the hospital on your affidavit sheet. An age-old debate is whether you should make it obvious by wearing your uniform to the exam. One school of thought says that you should not stand out. Yet feedback from those who wore their uniforms is emphatically favorable. You are so used to wearing your uniform anyway that it is a comforting familiarity. Most civilians and especially you feel stuffy and artificial in a business suit that is otherwise the necessary attire.

The uniform also lends a second-nature military bearing of extreme professionalism (e.g., ma'am, sir) that is not routinely bestowed on examiners. They relish this tremendous display of respect and professionalism. They cannot help but extend the same courtesy to you. Not only do they admire your devotion to duty, they also respect the additional challenges and hardships that you incur simply because you are a military physician. You will be taken aback, when ABOG dignitaries, as well as your examiners, will thank you for serving our country.

I believe that military bearing and courtesy also make the oral exam format more familiar. You seem to be able to bear the brunt of interrogation a little more easily than civilians. If you are not comfortable with your training experience alone, you can take a mock oral exam offered at the October meeting of the ACOG Armed Forces district.

In summary, I say, "Don't hide it, flaunt it!" Of course I need to disclose that I am a retired Army Colonel, but my career was with the National Guard and Reserves. I do know BOTH the civilian and military perspective. Having disclosed that, go with the winning tide and proudly acknowledge that you are in the military. Recall the impact of the first impression.

No doubt, a uniformed physician will make the ultimate first expression. After all, the adage, "You never get a second chance to make a great first impression," is posted in the entry to the AMEDD school hall at Ft. Sam Houston, Texas!

Appendix G

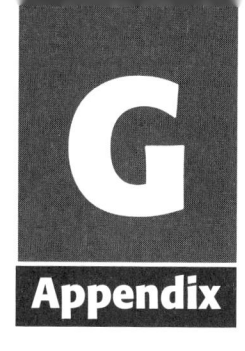

Case List Review

We have discussed throughout the book, the importance of having your case list reviewed. Of course, it is the most helpful BEFORE you turn it in on August 1. Your reviewers will pick up on not just the obvious, but equally important the subtleties that can really add up. Ideally you should have you case list reviewed in May and then in early-July after your first re-write.

The more reviews, the better. I recommend your referring MFM review the Obstetrics case list, your GYN Oncologist or FPM your Gynecology case list, and your Reproductive Endocrinologist your Office Practice. The specialists represent those of your examiners and are especially important to help you recapture the specialist, rather than the generalist perspective.

Given however, this is your *general* boards, I recommend you have some generalists look at any of the three sections. Furthermore, you want to have a stranger who is unfamiliar with your mode of practice, to give you a true unbiased picture. Finally, a non-medical person can pick up on typos and spelling errors.

Absolutely ALL of your reviewers should be clinicians. The practice of medicine is so dynamic, that even one who only recently stopped practicing will already be out of date. This exam most definitely will hold you to the latest standards. Furthermore, your reviewer must also be performing the same surgeries and procedures as you in order to provide the most contemporary and comprehensive suggestions. You can sure bet your examiner is the expert for those as well.

Prior to August 1, the reviews are targeted to helping you strategically organize the case list to put your best foot forward. After August 1, the case list is cast in stone, and subsequent reviews help you defend your case list.

If you would like me to review your case list, please contact me.

>Krishna Das, MD, FACOG
>(828) 606-6956
>(877) 222-6249
>krisdas@americasboardreview.com
>krisdas@morrisbb.net

Index

A

Abbreviations and acronyms, 185–186
ABOG (American Board of Obstetrics and Gynecology)
  ABOG-approved abbreviations, 54, 183–184
  address and Website, 187
  software, 189–190
Acceptance, notification of, 7
ACOG (American College of Obstetricians and Gynecologists)
  address and Website, 187
  Committee Opinions, 13
  Compendium, 13, 66–67, 76, 146, 149
  Precis, 12, 67
Acronyms and abbreviations, 185–186
Admission criteria, 30
American Board of Obstetrics and Gynecology. *See* ABOG
American College of Obstetricians and Gynecologists. *See* ACOG
Appearance. *See also* **Image enhancement**
  as first impression, 68
  image enhancement, 137
Application process, 5–8
Author address and Website, 218

B

Board review course, 15
Body language, 151

C

Candidate
  candidate's journey example, 161–174
  qualifications, 8
Case list
  acceptable abbreviations, 56
  appearance as first impression, 62, 68, 137–140
  appropriate Friedman Terminology example, 40, 64
  clinical summary extract example, 78–79
  color-coding in, 76
  column confusion example, 78, 80–81
  copies, 55–56
  critique, 77
  data collection, 31–33
  defense of, 67–77
  deidentification, 40, 55
  edited version example, 88
  editing of, 63–66
  format, 55–57
  fraudulent, 62
  gynecologic practice
    clinical summary example, 46
    gynecological categories, 42
    initial ABOG form entry, 47–48
    list of, 42
    pathologic diagnosis, 45
    pre-operative or admission diagnosis, 45–46
    sequential ordering, 56
  initial draft, 33

219

Case list *(continued...)*
   insufficient, carelessly prepared, 58
   "just right" case, 58, 82, 100
   key words in, 62
   lessons learned, 175–181
   logistics, 55
   management flow, 98–99
   obstetric practice
      clinical summary example, 41–42
      initial ABOG form entry, 41
      list of, 33–34
      obstetrical categories, 34–39
      red flag, 69
      sequential ordering, 40
      summary sheet, 68
   office practice
      categories, 49–50
      clinical summary example, 52–53
      column confusion, 50
      list of, 47
   organization, 27
   patient order consideration, 61
   peer review, 54
   poor outcome case, 62
   preparedness, 67
   purpose of, 67
   review, 217–218
   software, 189–190
   spelling and grammatical errors in, 75
   strategic organization, 57–63
   as study tool, 66–67
   styles, 53
   summary sheet, 200
   timetable, 25
   "too long" case, 59–60, 83–84
   too many patients per page, 87
   "too short" case, 59, 85–86
   working of cases, 61
Case of the day, 105
   failure of, 106
   format, 106–107
   overview, 105
Centers for Medicare and Medicaid Services (CMS), 3
Clothing, image enhancement, 138–139
CMS (Centers for Medicare & Medicaid Services), 3
Commercial software, 190
Committee Opinions, 13
Compendium, 13, 66–67, 76
CREOG (Council on Resident Education in Obstetrics and Gynecology), 1, 71

D
Database
   gynecologic, 205–209
   obstetric, 203–204
   office practice, 205–207
   personal, 196
Deadlines, 6
Deidentification, 40, 55
Disciplinary action, 62

F
Failure
   case of the day, 98
   of oral exam, 7–8
   test results, 185–187
Falsification of data, 8
Fast track milestone, 5–6, 22–24
Fellow
   fast track milestones, 23–24
   recommendations for, 237–238
First impression
   appearance, 65–66
   image enhancement, 165–168
Fraudulent case list, 60
Friedman terminology, 86

G
Gynecologics practice
   case list
      clinical summary example, 46
      gynecological categories, 42
      initial ABOG form entry, 47
      list of, 47
      pathologic diagnosis, 45
      pre-operative or admission diagnosis, 44
      sequential ordering, 46
   database setup, 205
   "hot topics" on oral exam, 117–118
   "know cold" topics, 118
   kodachromes on past exams, 101, 105

Index

H
Hairstyle, image enhancement, 139
Handshake, image enhancement, 140
HIPPA (Health Insurance Portability and Accounting Act of 1996), 166

I
Image enhancement
　accessories, 139
　appearance, 139
　clothing, 138–139
　color, 139
　first impression, 137
　hairstyle, 139
　handshake, 140
　oral communication, 140
　testmanship, 140
　voice quality, 140

K
Kodachromes, 101
　as case of the day, 105

L
Lessons learned, 175–181
License
　as requirement for exam, 6
　unrestricted, 7
Limitations, oral exam, 8
Litigation or investigation, 7

M
Maintenance of Certification (MOC), 13
Management flow (case list), 98–99
Milestones
　case list organization category, 25
　Fast track, 5–6, 22–24
　peer review category, 25–26
　study plan category, 26–27
　timing, 27
　Traditional track, 5–6, 21–22
Military personnel, recommendations for, 215–216
MOC (Maintenance of Certification), 13
Mock oral examination, 26–27, 133–136

N–O
Notification of acceptance, 7

Obstetrics practice
　Case list
　　clinical summary example, 41–42
　　common complications, recommended listings and treatment options, 38
　　diagnosis criteria, 40
　　HIPPA, 166
　　initial ABOG form entry, 41
　　list of, 34–36
　　obstetrical categories, 34–36
　　red flag, 69
　　sequential ordering, 40
　　summary sheet, 200–202
　database setup, 203–204
　"hot topics" on oral exam, 128–131
　"know cold" topics, 118–128
　kodachromes on past exams, 105
Office practice
　Case list
　　categories, 49–50
　　clinical summary example, 53
　　column confusion, 50
　　list of, 53
　database setup, 205–209
　"hot topics" on oral exam, 130–131
　"know cold" topics, 123–128
Oral examination
　body language during, 151
　conduct, 147–151
　content, 144–147
　end of, 153
　evaluation criteria, 146
　examiner alerts, 146–147
　eye contact during, 138, 151
　failure, 10–12, 157
　format, 176
　impact of, 3
　limitations, 8
　location of, 141
　mock, 26
　points for style, 151–152
　preparation for, timetable
　　day before, 142–143
　　day of, 143–144

Oral examination *(continued...)*
    repeat exam, 153
    scope of, 9–10
    suspension from, 62
    time length, 145
    written exam *versus*, 1–3

P

Pass rate, 10, 156
Patient scenarios. *See* Case of the day
Peer review
    case list, 54
    milestone category, 20
Policy Statements, 13
Practice Bulletins, 13
Precis, 12, 67
Professional misbehavior, 8
PROLOG (Personal Review of Learning on Obstetrics and Gynecology), 12

R

References
    Committee Opinions, 13
    Compendium, 13
    Policy Statements, 13
    Practice Bulletins, 13
    Precis, 12
    PROLOG (Personal Review of Learning on Obstetrics and Gynecology), 12
    Technology Assessments, 13
Requirements to sit for exam, 7
Review courses, 14–15
    agenda, 17
    board, 15
    cost, 16
    length of, 19–20
    necessity of, 14
    when to attend, 14–15

S

Scope of exam, 9–10
Software
    ABOG, 189–190
    commercial, 190
    products, 192–193

Structured cases. *See* Case of the day
Study tools
    case list as, 66
    colleagues as, 134
    "hot topics," 128–131
    "know cold" topics, 118–128
    lessons learned, 203–207
    mock oral exam, 133–136
    perfect practice concept, 136
    practicing out loud, 134
    priority of, 11–12
    procrastination, 31–32
    references, 12–13
    review courses, 14–18
    review of other candidate case list, 133
    study plan, 133
    tutorial courses, 18–20
    weekly/monthly, 117–118
Summary sheet, 74

T

Technology Assessments, 13
Test results
    fail, 157–159
    pass rate, 215
    pass requirements, 155–156
Traditional track milestone, 5–6, 20–21
Tutorial courses, 18–20, 179
Tutoring, 15

V–W

Voice quality, image enhancement, 140

Website
    ABOG, 5–7, 9, 217
    ACOG, 216
    author, 189
Written *versus* oral exam, 1–3